WITHDRAWN

Magic Menus

for People with Diabetes
2nd edition

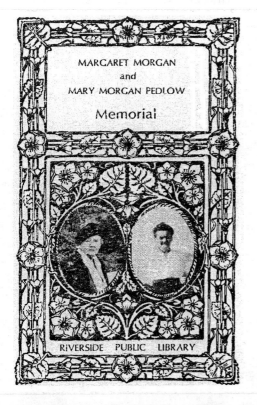

D0391283

American Diabetes Association

Cure • Care • Commitment℠

Director, Book Publishing, John Fedor; *Associate Director, Consumer Books,* Sherrye L. Landrum; *Editor,* Laurie Guffey; *Production Manager,* Peggy M. Rote; *Composition,* Tom Suzuki, Inc.; *Nutritional Analysis,* Nutritional Computing Concepts, Inc.; *Cover Design,* Koncept Inc.; *Cover Photography,* John Burwell, Burwell/Burwell Photography; *Cover Food Stylist,* Lisa Cherkasky; *Printer,* Transcontinental Printing.

Printed Canada
1 3 5 7 9 10 8 6 4 2

The suggestions and information contained in this publication are generally consistent with the *Clinical Practice Recommendations* and other policies of the American Diabetes Association, but they do not represent the policy or position of the Association or any of its boards or committees. Reasonable steps have been taken to ensure the accuracy of the information presented. However, the American Diabetes Association cannot ensure the safety or efficacy of any product or service described in this publication. Individuals are advised to consult a physician or other appropriate health care professional before undertaking any diet or exercise program or taking any medication referred to in this publication. Professionals must use and apply their own professional judgment, experience, and training and should not rely solely on the information contained in this publication before prescribing any diet, exercise, or medication. The American Diabetes Association—its officers, directors, employees, volunteers, and members—assumes no responsibility or liability for personal or other injury, loss, or damage that may result from the suggestions or information in this publication.

∞ The paper in this publication meets the requirements of the ANSI Standard Z39.48-1992 (permanence of paper).

ADA titles may be purchased for business or promotional use or for special sales. To purchase this book in large quantities, or for custom editions of this book with your logo, contact Lee Romano Sequeira, Special Sales & Promotions, at the address below, or at LRomano@diabetes.org or 703-299-2046.

American Diabetes Association
1701 North Beauregard Street
Alexandria, Virginia 22311

Library of Congress Cataloging-in-Publication Data
Magic Menus : for people with diabetes.—2nd ed.
    p. cm.
Includes index.
ISBN 1-58040-173-2 (pbk. : alk. Paper)
1. Diabetes—Diet therapy—Recipes. I. American Diabetes Association.

RC662.M333 2003
641.5'6314—dc21   2002043720

Contents

Acknowledgments iv

Introduction 1

The Six Food Groups..3

Guidelines for Good Nutrition 5

How to Use This Book...8

Breakfast..15

Lunch 51

Dinner 99

Snacks...193

Nutritional Analyses..211

Index 243

Acknowledgments

The meals in *Magic Menus* were originally created for the *Month of Meals* series of books by committees of volunteers from the Council on Nutritional Science and Metabolism of the Professional Section of the American Diabetes Association. Committee members, for one or more of the five books, included the following registered dietitians: Marion Franz, MS, RD; Nancy Cooper, RD; Lois Babione, RD; Anne Daly, MS, RD, CDE; Robin Ann Williams, MA, RD, CDE; Marti Chitwood, RD, CDE; Susan L. Thom, RD, CDE; Ruth Kangas, RD, CDE; Carolyn Leontos, MS, RD, CDE; Joyce Cooper, MA, RD; Deborah Fillman, MS, RD, CDE; and Dennis Gordon, RD, CDE. Nutritional analyses were provided by Madelyn Wheeler.

Most of the recipes were developed by the committee members who worked on *Month of Meals* or were published in *Diabetes Forecast*, the American Diabetes Association's monthly magazine on healthy living with diabetes. The exceptions are noted below.

The recipes for French Dressing, Sloppy Joes, Chicken Cacciatore, Oven-Fried Fish, Crisp Red Cabbage, Meat Loaf, and Gazpacho appear in *American Diabetes Association/American Dietetic Association Family Cookbook, Volume I*, © 1980 by the American Diabetes Association, Inc., and The American Dietetic Association, Inc., and are used with permission of the publisher, Prentice Hall Press.

The recipes for Crunchy Granola, Cheesy Grits, Apple-Raisin Muffins, Fluffy High-Fiber Low-Fat Pancakes, Noodle Supreme Salad, Black Bean Soup, Chicken Tacos, Oven-Fried Chicken, Vegetarian Lasagna, and Herbed Pork Kabobs appear in *American Diabetes Association/American Dietetic Association Family Cookbook, Volume II*, © 1984 by the American Diabetes Association, Inc., and The American Dietetic Association, Inc., and are used with permission of the publisher, Prentice Hall Press.

For information on ordering *Magic Menus* or any of the *Month of Meals* books, call 1-800-232-6733. For information on joining the American Diabetes Association (ADA), call 1-800-806-7801.

People with diabetes can eat almost anything—including packaged foods, such as frozen entrees—as long as their overall diet is well balanced. As a convenient aid to readers who want fast yet healthy meal choices, *Magic Menus* includes some brand names or product names. The use of selected brand names does not mean that they are the only brands suitable for people with diabetes. Although we tried to be sure that these packaged foods met the calorie levels of individual menus, the ADA does not endorse these products or guarantee that they are appropriate for all people with diabetes. You are encouraged to read food labels carefully and to consult with a registered dietitian to determine whether a food fits into your meal plan.

Introduction

Most cookbooks give you lots of recipes and only a few suggestions for combining them into a day's meals. When you find a recipe you like, you still must choose other foods to round out the meal. People with diabetes have the added challenge of counting the carbohydrate in the meal so they'll know what effect it will have on their blood glucose level. A simple but unexciting solution is to eat the same things day after day. A better solution is found in this book and the other books in the ADA's *Month of Meals* series. The menus are counted and balanced for you. Just cook and eat!

Magic Menus will help you choose healthy foods to make up your daily menus easily. You will find many menus that can be prepared quickly, menus built around favorite family dishes, meatless menus, and menus emphasizing low-fat and high-fiber foods. For people who cook for just one or two, most of these recipes can be prepared and then divided into serving sizes and frozen for quick, no-fuss future meals.

There are complete menus for breakfast, lunch, dinner, and snacks. One day's menu selections—breakfast, lunch, dinner, and a snack—provides approximately 1,500 calories. Directions are given for adjusting the menus to other calorie levels. Each day's menus will provide about 45–50 percent of your calories from carbohydrate, 20 percent from protein, and about 30 percent from fat. Look on page 211 for complete nutritional analyses for each recipe.

If you're counting carbohydrate (carb), use the bold number under the menu number. That is the total grams of carb in the menu. Knowing your carb totals for each meal and snack and keeping these totals consistent have a great effect on your blood glucose levels! (For more information on carb counting, see page 10.)

These menus will help you

■ **Eat a variety of foods.** Eating a wide variety of different foods helps you get all the essential vitamins, minerals, and nutrients your body needs. Variety also helps keep your interest so that your diet doesn't become boring. With *Magic Menus,* you can mix and match thousands of combinations of breakfasts, lunches, and dinners.

■ **Maintain a healthy weight.** *Magic Menus* allows you to add and subtract snacks to get just the right number of calories for you to achieve and maintain a healthy body weight.

■ **Choose a meal plan low in fat, saturated fat, and cholesterol.** The meals in *Magic Menus* average less than 300 milligrams of cholesterol per day and less than 30 percent total fat. These menus emphasize low-fat foods.

■ **Eat plenty of vegetables, fruits, and whole-grain products.** These foods not only add variety to your diet, but they also can be an important source of fiber. Unrefined foods are close in form to what Mother Nature gives us, and the closer to the source, the better.

■ **Use sugars only in moderation.** It's okay to eat sugar as part of a balanced meal. But you still need to watch empty calories and the amount of carbohydrate you eat. That's why most of these recipes are low in sugar. Instead of sugar, you can also use sugar substitutes that have essentially no calories.

■ **Watch sodium levels in processed foods.** While packaged and fast foods are convenient, they can sometimes be high in added salt. If you need to watch your sodium intake, check package labels carefully. In general, though, sodium recommendations for people with diabetes (without hypertension) are the same as those for the general population. (If you have diabetes and hypertension, try to stay below 2,400 mg of sodium per day.)

2

The Six Food Groups

The menus in *Magic Menus* have been developed using a meal-planning system that divides foods into six groups: Starch, Meat and Meat Substitutes, Vegetables, Fruit, Milk, and Fat. Foods are placed into one group or another based on their nutrient makeup—carbohydrate, protein, fat, and calories.

Starch. This group includes whole grains (brown rice, bulgur wheat, wheat berries, oats, barley), cereal, pasta, rice, breads, starchy vegetables (potatoes, corn, lima beans, and winter squashes such as acorn and spaghetti), crackers, desserts, and many snack-type foods.

Meat and Meat Substitutes. This group includes beef, pork, lamb, veal, poultry, fish, seafood, eggs, tofu, cheese, cottage cheese, and peanut butter. Foods are then divided into very lean, lean, medium-fat, and high-fat choices.

Vegetables. The vegetable group is made up of nonstarchy vegetables, either raw or cooked, such as broccoli, asparagus, green beans, cabbage, carrots, salad greens, onions, tomatoes, and summer squashes like crookneck and zucchini.

Fruit. This group includes all varieties of fruit—fresh, frozen, canned, and dried—as well as fruit juices.

Milk. Included here are milk, yogurt, and buttermilk.

Fat. You have obvious fats like margarine, butter, cooking oils, mayonnaise, and salad dressings plus other high-fat foods like avocados, olives, nuts and seeds, bacon, sour cream, and cream cheese.

For a complete listing of foods and serving sizes in the six food groups, see *Exchange Lists for Meal Planning*, available from the American Diabetes Association or The American

Dietetic Association, or contact a registered dietitian. If you plan to adjust the meals in this book (see pages 8–11), you'll need to know what nutrients are in a serving from each of the food groups. This information is found in *Exchange Lists for Meal Planning.*

Food Group	Calories	Per Serving Carbo-hydrate (grams)	Protein (grams)	Fat (grams)
Starch	80	15	3	trace
Meat and Substitutes				
Lean	55	0	7	3
Medium Fat	75	0	7	5
High Fat	100	0	0	0
Vegetables	25	5	2	0
Fruit	60	15	0	0
Milk				
Fat Free	90	12	8	trace
Low Fat (1%)	102	12	8	3
Whole	150	12	8	8
Fat	45	0	0	5

Guidelines for Good Nutrition

Good nutrition comes from eating a variety of foods. No single food will supply all of the nutrients your body needs; therefore, you should eat from each of the food groups every day. It's also a good idea to vary the foods you eat within each food group from day to day. For example, eat an apple or orange from time to time instead of always having a banana. Here are some more guidelines to healthy food choices.

Eat less fat. To cut back on fat, you can

■ Eat smaller portions of meat.

■ Eat fish and poultry (without the skin) more often.

■ Choose lean cuts of red meat.

■ Prepare meats by broiling, roasting, or baking instead of frying. Trim off all fat before cooking and remove the skin from poultry before eating it.

■ Avoid adding fat in cooking.

■ Avoid fried foods.

■ Avoid sauces or gravy.

■ Eat fewer high-fat foods, such as cold cuts, bacon, sausage, hot dogs, butter, mayonnaise, nuts, salad dressing, lard, and solid shortening.

■ Drink fat-free or low-fat (1%) milk.

■ Eat less ice cream, cheese, sour cream, cream, whole milk, and other high-fat dairy products. Use low-fat or fat-free yogurt or low-fat cottage cheese instead of sour cream. Use low-fat cheeses.

Eat more high-fiber foods. *Magic Menus* includes lots of high-fiber foods—fruits, vegetables, and whole-grain products—in the meals. In general,

■ Eat more whole-grain breads, cereals, and crackers. Eat more dried beans, peas, and lentils, too.

■ Eat high-fiber foods, such as oat bran, brown rice, wild rice, barley, and bulgur.

■ Eat more vegetables (raw and cooked). You can have large servings of raw, nonstarchy vegetables when called for in a menu, which may include salad greens, carrot or celery sticks, tomatoes, cucumbers, green peppers, radishes, and the like.

■ Eat whole fruit instead of drinking fruit juice.

In this book, you may:

■ Use commercial (canned, dried, or frozen) or homemade soups with these menus, but note that they are usually high in sodium, so choose reduced-fat and reduced-sodium varieties.

■ Use no-sugar or low-sugar fruit spreads (jams or jellies). Limit yourself to 1 to 2 teaspoons (less than 20 calories) per serving.

■ Use 1 tablespoon of regular salad dressing or 2 tablespoons of reduced-fat salad dressing interchangeably. Salad dressings that contain less than 6 calories per tablespoon can be used more liberally.

■ Have raw vegetables on some menus, which can include salad greens and moderate servings of carrot or celery sticks, tomatoes, cucumbers, green peppers, radishes, and the like.

■ Use butter-flavored granules, such as Butter Buds or Molly McButter, to season vegetables, potatoes, rice, or noodles.

■ Add your choice of calorie-free beverages, such as coffee, hot or iced tea, mineral water, diet sodas, and sugar-free flavored seltzers.

■ Measure meat portions after cooking. Four ounces of uncooked meat shrinks to about 3 ounces (about the size of a deck of cards) after cooking.

■ Season recipes with your favorite spices. Try basil, dill, lemon pepper, paprika, fresh herbs, and fresh garlic or garlic powder. Be sure to choose low-salt varieties when mixtures are purchased.

The recipes in this book use these standard abbreviations:

Tbsp = tablespoon
tsp = teaspoon
oz = ounce
lb = pound
qt = quart

How to Use This Book

Magic Menus allows you to choose the calorie level that best meets your needs. First, you need to know how many calories you require daily. The best way to do this is to meet with a registered dietitian or certified diabetes educator, who can design a meal plan with the right number of calories for your nutritional needs.

BASIC MEAL PLAN: 1,500 CALORIES A DAY

Each breakfast, lunch, and dinner in *Magic Menus* has about the same number of calories as the other breakfasts, or lunches, or dinners, so you can mix and match them to suit your own tastes. One day's breakfast, lunch, and dinner add up to about 1,350 calories. By adding two 60-calorie snacks OR one 125-calorie snack, your daily total will be 1,500 calories—the Basic Meal Plan. Choose any menus you like. All the portions on the menus are for one person, so you can have everything listed.

If you need more or fewer calories than this, no problem. Adjusting meals to meet your requirements is easy.

BASIC MEAL PLAN PLUS

If you are following a meal plan that allows you 1,800 calories a day, use the chart on the next page to adjust the Basic Meal Plan.

First, choose any menu in *Magic Menus* that you want. Then, move down the 1,800-calorie column and follow the directions. Breakfast, lunch, and dinner are the same as in the Basic Meal Plan. The extra calories you need will come from snacks—a 125-calorie morning snack, a 125-calorie afternoon snack, and a 170-calorie evening snack.

The chart also shows you how to reach a 2,100-calorie meal plan. You may want to alter this plan to meet your needs if you are pregnant or breastfeeding.

BASIC MEAL PLAN MINUS

If you are following a meal plan of 1,200 calories a day, use the chart on page 11 to adjust the Basic Meal Plan. To meet your body's nutritional needs, you need to eat at least 1,200 calories a day.

8

Basic Meal Plan Plus

Meal	1,500 Calories (Basic Meal Plan)	1,800 Calories	2,100 Calories
Breakfast	Total calories: 350	Same as Basic Meal Plan Total calories: 350	Add 1 Starch OR 1 Meat to the Basic Meal Plan Total calories: 450
Morning Snack		Add 1 125-calorie snack Total calories: 125	Add 1 60-calorie snack Total calories: 60
Lunch	Total calories: 450	Same as Basic Meal Plan Total calories: 450	Add 1 Starch AND 1 Fat to the Basic Meal Plan Total calories: 575
Afternoon Snack		Add 1 125-calorie snack Total calories: 125	Add 1 125-calorie snack Total calories: 125
Dinner	Total calories: 550	Same as Basic Meal Plan Total calories: 550	Add 1 Starch AND 1 Milk to the Basic Meal Plan Total calories: 720
Evening Snack	2 60-calorie snacks OR 1 125-calorie snack Total calories: 125	Add 1 170-calorie snack Total calories: 170	Add 1 170-calorie snack Total calories: 170

First, choose any menu in *Magic Menus* that you want. Then, move down the 1,200-calorie column and follow the directions: Take away 1 Starch or 1 Milk from breakfast in the Basic Meal Plan. Take away 1 Fruit at lunch from the Basic Meal Plan. Take away 1 Fat at dinner from the Basic Meal Plan. There are no snacks in the 1,200-calorie meal plan. This chart also shows you how to reach a 1,350-calorie meal plan.

CARBOHYDRATE COUNTING
The number of carbohydrate (carb) grams is listed on each menu.

WHY COUNT CARB?
Why should you count the grams of carb you eat? Because it is the carb in food that raises your blood glucose levels! And it raises them in predictable ways. If you eat about the same amount of carb at each meal and snack, chances are your blood glucose levels will settle into a steady pattern, giving you greater glucose control and a much-reduced risk of diabetes complications. You can also add new foods to your meal plan if you count the grams of carb in them—then you just substitute one carbohydrate-containing food for the other.

HOW TO COUNT CARB
First, you need to know the number of carb grams in the food you're eating. If you're following the exchange meal planning system, each starch, fruit, and milk serving has about 15 grams of carbohydrate. A vegetable serving has about 5 grams of carbohydrate. The carb choices meal planning system also has 15 grams of carbohydrate per serving.

If you look at the Nutrition Facts on a food label, you'll find the carb grams per serving listed under Total Carbohydrate. (Be careful not to confuse the gram weight of the food, listed after the serving size, with grams of Total Carbohydrate.) Under Total Carbohydrate are Sugars and Dietary Fiber. Ignore the Sugars because they are included in the Total Carb. But if you eat more than 5 grams of fiber, you can subtract it from the total carb count (another reason why high-fiber foods are a healthy bonus for you).

Next, you need to know how many grams of carb to eat at each meal, based on your diabetes treatment plan (exercise, diabetes pills, and/or insulin). Most adults need about 60–75 grams of carb at each meal.

Basic Meal Plan Minus

Meal	1,200 Calories	1,350 Calories	1,500 Calories (Basic Meal Plan)
Breakfast	Take away 1 Starch OR 1 Milk from Basic Meal Plan Total calories: 270	Same as Basic Meal Plan Total calories: 350	Total calories: 350
Morning Snack			
Lunch	Take away 1 Fruit from Basic Meal Plan Total calories: 390	Same as Basic Meal Plan Total calories: 450	Total calories: 450
Afternoon Snack			
Dinner	Take away 1 Fat from Basic Meal Plan Total calories: 505	Same as Basic Meal Plan Total calories: 550	Total calories: 550
Evening Snack			2 60-calorie snacks OR 1 125-calorie snack Total calories: 125

Sample Meal Plan 1

Here's how to adjust the Basic Meal Plan (1,500 calories) for about 1,200 calories.

Meal	Calories		
Breakfast			
(Plus or minus)	350		
−1 Starch serving(s)			
# (type of serving)	−80	Subtotal	270
Lunch			
(Plus or minus)	450		
−1 Fruit serving(s)			
# (type of serving)	−60	Subtotal	390
Dinner			
(Plus or minus)	550		
−1 Fat serving(s)			
# (type of serving)	−45	Subtotal	505

Total Daily Calories   1,165

It's important to measure your serving sizes. A bigger serving has more carb. Add up your carb totals at each meal, and try to keep your totals within your range to get the benefits of better blood glucose control. (For more information, check out ADA's Complete Guide to Carbohydrate Counting.)

How This Book Helps

Simply check the carb gram total under each menu number. To keep your daily totals consistent, choose meals and snacks that add up to your desired number. For example, on Monday choose Breakfast 21, Lunch 12, Dinner 17, and 60-calorie Snack 5 for a daily total of 182 carb grams. The next day, eat Breakfast 10, Lunch 9, Dinner 26, and 60-calorie Snack 3 for a total of 214 carb grams. Knowing the carb totals for every meal really helps you stay consistent from day to day!

12

Sample Meal Plan 2

Here's how to adjust the Basic Meal Plan (1,500 calories) for about 2,200 calories.

Meal   **Calories**

Breakfast
(Plus or minus)   __350__
+1_____ __Starch__ serving(s)
(type of serving)   __+80__   Subtotal __430__

Lunch
(Plus or minus)   __450__
+1_____ __Fat__ serving(s)
(type of serving)   __+60__

+1_____ __Fruit__ serving(s)
(type of serving)   __+45__   Subtotal __555__

Dinner
(Plus or minus)   __550__
+1_____ __Starch__ serving(s)
(type of serving)   __+80__

+1_____ __Meat__ serving(s)
(type of serving)   __+75__

+1_____ __Fat__ serving(s)
(type of serving)   __+45__   Subtotal __750__

Snacks (Morning, Afternoon, and/or Evening)
(Plus or minus)   __125__
+2_____ __Starch__ serving(s)
(type of serving)   __160__

+2_____ __Milk or Meat__ serving(s)
(type of serving)   __180__   Subtotal __465__

                     Total Daily Calories __2,200__

Your Meal Plan

Meal	Calories	Carb
Breakfast (Plus or minus)	_____	_____
_____ _____ serving(s) # (type of serving)	_____	_____
	Subtotal	Subtotal
Lunch (Plus or minus)	_____	_____
_____ _____ serving(s) # (type of serving)	_____	_____
_____ _____ serving(s) # (type of serving)	_____	_____
	Subtotal	Subtotal
Dinner (Plus or minus)	_____	_____
_____ _____ serving(s) # (type of serving)	_____	_____
_____ _____ serving(s) # (type of serving)	_____	_____
_____ _____ serving(s) # (type of serving)	_____	_____
	Subtotal	Subtotal
Snacks (Plus or minus)	_____	_____
_____ _____ serving(s) # (type of serving)	_____	_____
_____ _____ serving(s) # (type of serving)	_____	_____
	Subtotal	Subtotal
	Total Daily Calories	**Total Daily Carbs**

*B*reakfast

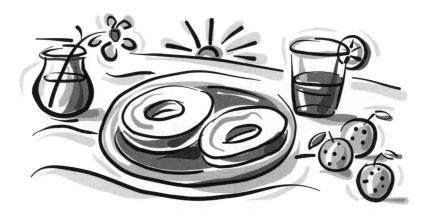

Each breakfast in this section has
about 350 calories and includes
2 starch servings
1 fruit serving
1 fat-free milk serving
1 fat serving

Average Fat: 5 grams

Average Carbohydrate: 57 grams

Average Protein: 14 grams

Some menus have 1 meat serving
instead of 1 fat-free milk or 1
starch serving.

No-Fuss Mornings

1

56g carb

¾ cup cornflakes with
1 cup fat-free milk
1 slice whole-wheat toast with
1 tsp margarine
1 cup cantaloupe cubes

2

66g carb

1 round toaster waffle
1¼ cups fresh strawberries
½ cup fat-free plain yogurt
¼ cup Grape-Nuts cereal
½ cup fat-free milk

Top waffle with mixture of strawberries and yogurt. Sprinkle with Grape-Nuts.

3

41g carb

1 slice whole-wheat toast with
1 tsp 100% fruit spread and
1 Tbsp reduced-fat margarine
1 egg or ¼ cup egg substitute, scrambled
   with nonstick cooking spray
½ grapefruit
1 cup fat-free milk

4

51g carb

1 cup cooked oatmeal with
Dash cinnamon and brown sugar substitute
    (optional)
1 Tbsp raisins
¼ cup unsweetened applesauce
1 cup fat-free milk

5

51g carb

2 slices French toast with
1 Tbsp reduced-fat margarine or 1 tsp
    regular margarine and
2 Tbsp sugar-free syrup (optional)
½ cup unsweetened applesauce with
Dash cinnamon
1 cup fat-free milk

*Dip 2 slices of bread in beaten egg. Brown on both sides in a
pan coated with nonstick cooking spray.*

6

55g carb

1 slice whole-wheat toast with
2 tsp 100% fruit spread and
1 tsp margarine
1 cup fat-free artificially sweetened fruit-
    flavored yogurt topped with
3 Tbsp wheat germ and
½ small banana, sliced

59g carb

2 4-inch pancakes with
¾ cup blueberries, fresh or frozen,
    unsweetened
1 tsp. margarine
1 cup fat-free or low-fat (1%) milk

To make a blueberry sauce, microwave blueberries briefly, until they thicken to desired consistency.

55g carb

1 English muffin with
1 tsp 100% fruit spread and
1 tsp margarine
1 serving Strawberry Blender Drink

Combine 1 cup fat-free or low-fat (1%) milk and 1¼ cups strawberries, fresh or frozen, no sugar added, in a blender and blend until smooth and creamy.

43g carb

1 poached egg
1 whole-wheat English muffin with
1 tsp margarine
½ large pear

10

61g carb

1½ cups puffed rice with
1 cup fat-free or low-fat (1%) milk
½ English muffin with
½ Tbsp peanut butter
1 small nectarine

11

56g carb

½ cup cooked grits
1 slice whole-wheat toast
1 Tbsp reduced-fat margarine
1 tsp low-sugar fruit spread
½ cup orange juice
1 cup fat-free milk

12

56g carb

Breakfast Tortilla:
    ½ cup egg substitute, scrambled with
    2 Tbsp chopped onion and
    2 Tbsp chopped green pepper and
    2 Tbsp salsa, wrapped in
    2 6-inch soft tortillas
1 kiwi fruit

1 cup cooked kasha, oat groats, brown rice, or wheat berries with
2 Tbsp raisins and
2 Tbsp walnuts, chopped
Dash cinnamon and sugar substitute (optional)
1 cup fat-free or low-fat (1%) milk

13

60g carb

Whole grains require 30–45 minutes of cooking. To speed up breakfast, cook cereal the night before, then heat up in the morning. Other alternatives are to pour hot water over grains the night before to soften them and save time the next morning or to cook them overnight in a slow cooker or Crockpot.

1 2-oz pumpernickel bagel with
1½ Tbsp low-fat cream cheese
3 medium stewed prunes
1 cup fat-free or low-fat (1%) milk

14

66g carb

15

50g carb

Strawberry Shortcake:
1 3-inch biscuit
1¼ cups sliced strawberries
1 cup fat-free milk
Sugar substitute as desired

Split biscuit and place half in a bowl. Cover with half of strawberries, then top with other half of biscuit. Cover with remaining strawberries and pour milk over biscuit and strawberries.

16

66g carb

¼ cup Grape-Nuts cereal in
½ cup low-fat artificially sweetened lemon yogurt with
¾ cup water-packed mandarin oranges, drained
1 piece whole-wheat toast with
1 tsp margarine

17

54g carb

Cinnamon Tortilla Pocket:
2 6-inch tortillas filled with
¼ cup ricotta cheese blended with
½ packet sugar substitute and
¼ tsp cinnamon
¾ cup fresh pineapple, mango, kiwi,
banana, and/or papaya

Spread mixture down middle of tortilla; fold four sides over into a square and microwave on low for 30 seconds until warm.

18

41g carb

2 Cheese Cornucopias:
2 slices bread
1 oz low-fat cheese, grated
1 tsp soft margarine
½ cup orange juice
1 cup fat-free milk

Trim crusts from bread and sprinkle bread with cheese. Fold each slice in half and secure with a toothpick. Spread top with margarine. Place on tray in toaster oven at 350 degrees until brown, about 10 minutes. Remove toothpicks to serve.

Bacon and Egg Sandwich:
    2 slices high-fiber bread, toasted
    1 egg, cooked in nonstick pan
    1 strip bacon, cooked crisp
1 medium tangelo
½ cup fat-free milk

19

44g carb

Breakfast Parfait:
    1 cup fat-free artificially sweetened
      vanilla yogurt
    4 pecan halves, chopped
    1 small banana, sliced
    3 Tbsp wheat germ
    3 graham crackers (2½-inch squares)

Layer yogurt, pecans, banana, and wheat germ in a parfait glass.

20

58g carb

Commuter Breakfast:
    1 Tbsp peanut butter
    1 cup fat-free plain yogurt
    1 small banana
    3 or 4 ice cubes (optional)
    Sugar substitute, if desired
    ½ cup All-Bran cereal

Blend all ingredients except cereal in a blender. Pour in mug, then top with cereal.

21

60g carb

2 cups puffed kasha
6 dry-roasted almonds
¾ cup blueberries
55g carb 1 cup fat-free milk

2 frozen waffles topped with
½ cup unsweetened applesauce
1 oz Canadian bacon
47g carb 2 Tbsp sugar-free syrup

½ cup cooked oatmeal with
3 Tbsp wheat germ and
6 dry-roasted almonds, chopped, and
1 small banana, sliced, and
54g carb Cinnamon to taste
1 cup fat-free milk

25

68g carb

1 **Sugar-Free Blueberry Muffin**
½ cup bran flakes with
1 cup fat-free or low-fat (1%) milk
½ cup fresh pineapple chunks

Sugar-Free Blueberry Muffins

Yield: 12 muffins / Serving size: 1 muffin

INGREDIENTS

1 cup blueberries, picked over and rinsed
1¾ cups plus 2 tsp all-purpose flour
1 Tbsp baking powder
¼ tsp nutmeg
¼ tsp cinnamon
2 eggs
¼ cup canola oil
¾ cup orange juice
1 tsp grated lemon or orange rind

METHOD

1. Preheat oven to 400 degrees. Spray muffin tin with nonstick cooking spray or line with baking cups.
2. Lightly coat the blueberries with 2 tsp flour by shaking together in a paper bag.
3. In a large bowl, stir together 1¾ cups flour, baking powder, nutmeg, and cinnamon.
4. In a small bowl, beat the eggs lightly. Add oil, orange juice, and grated rind.
5. Add the liquid to the dry mixture and stir gently. Before the two mixtures are fully combined, fold in the blueberries.
6. Fill each muffin cup about two-thirds full. Bake 20–25 minutes.

26

1 cinnamon-raisin bagel with
¼ cup **Ricotta Cheese Spread**
½ cup orange juice

56g carb

Ricotta Cheese Spread

Yield: 1 serving / Serving size: ¼ cup

INGREDIENTS
¼ cup part-skim ricotta cheese
1 pkt. sugar substitute
⅛ tsp vanilla (or other flavoring)
Dash cinnamon

METHOD
1. Mix first three ingredients together.
2. Spread on bagel halves. Sprinkle with cinnamon.
3. Heat under broiler until hot, about 1–2 minutes.

27

54g carb

1 serving **Easy Spud Breakfast**
1 slice whole-grain toast
1 tsp reduced-calorie margarine
¾ cup mixed berries

Easy Spud Breakfast

Yield: 2 servings / Serving size: ½ recipe

INGREDIENTS

1 large baked potato with skin
¼ cup chopped onions
¼ cup chopped green or red peppers
1 oz lean ham, chopped
1 large egg, beaten
2 Tbsp shredded reduced-fat cheddar cheese
Fresh or dried parsley

METHOD

1. Preheat oven to 400 degrees.
2. Slice baked potato in half the long way. Scoop out one-third of the potato pulp (save for another meal). Set shells on a microwave-safe dish.
3. Spray a nonstick skillet with vegetable spray and sauté onions and peppers for about 5 minutes or until soft.
4. Add ham and sauté another 1–2 minutes. Add the beaten egg and cook until egg is done. Add salt and pepper to taste.
5. Fill each potato half with egg mixture. Top with grated cheese. Bake 5 minutes. Garnish with parsley.

2 Scones
1 Tbsp reduced-calorie margarine
½ cup pineapple juice
1 cup fat-free milk

28

58g carb

Scones

Yield: 16 scones / Serving size: 1 scone

INGREDIENTS

3 Tbsp reduced-fat margarine
1½ cups all-purpose flour
½ cup whole-wheat flour
1½ tsp baking powder
½ tsp baking soda
1 pkt. sugar substitute suitable for baking
¼–½ tsp salt (optional)
½ cup fat-free milk
¼ cup dark raisins or currants
¼ tsp orange peel

METHOD

1. Preheat oven to 450 degrees.
2. In food processor or with pastry blender, mix margarine and flours until the mixture resembles coarse crumbs. Stir in baking powder, baking soda, sugar substitute, and salt to taste.
3. Stir in milk until dry ingredients are moistened. Stir in raisins and orange peel.
4. Gather dough into a ball. Roll out on a lightly floured board to ½-inch thickness. Cut into rounds using a 2½-inch cookie cutter. Place on cookie sheet well coated with cooking spray.
5. Bake 7–10 minutes or until lightly browned.

2 **Graham Pudding Sandwiches**
1 small orange
1 cup fat-free milk

29

54g carb

Graham Pudding Sandwiches

Yield: 32 sandwiches / Serving size: 1 sandwich

INGREDIENTS

1 pkg. sugar-free chocolate instant pudding, prepared
½ cup natural peanut butter
64 graham cracker squares
cinnamon

METHOD

1. Prepare pudding according to package directions. Mix in
   ½ cup peanut butter.
2. Spread 1 Tbsp mixture on 1 graham cracker square and
   top with another graham cracker square. Place on foil-
   lined cookie sheet and freeze. Eat frozen or slightly
   thawed.

1 small plain muffin with
2 tsp 100% fruit spread
1 cup **Breakfast Blender Drink**

60g carb

Breakfast Blender Drink

Yield: 1 serving / Serving size: 1 cup

INGREDIENTS

1 cup fat-free milk
½ large banana, frozen and sliced
3 Tbsp wheat germ
½ tsp vanilla

METHOD

1. Combine all ingredients in blender and blend until smooth and creamy.
2. To freeze a banana, peel and place in a zippered plastic bag. Place in freezer for at least 8 hours.

31

47g carb

⅓ cup **Crunchy Granola**
1 cup vegetable juice
1 cup fat-free milk

Crunchy Granola

Yield: 16 servings / Serving size: ⅓ cup

INGREDIENTS
3½ cups rolled oats
½ cup wheat germ
½ cup shredded unsweetened coconut
¼ cup sesame seeds
¼ cup sliced almonds
¼ cup sunflower or millet seeds
¼ cup honey
¼ cup canola oil
1 Tbsp vanilla
½ cup raisins

METHOD
1. Preheat oven to 250 degrees.
2. Mix all ingredients except raisins together with electric mixer. Spread evenly on 2 baking sheets with edges. Bake until golden brown (45–60 minutes).
3. Turn and stir after 30 minutes.
4. Remove from oven and add raisins. Cool and store in plastic bag.

1 cup **Cheesy Grits**
½ grapefruit

46g carb

Cheesy Grits

Yield: 2 servings / Serving size: 1 cup

INGREDIENTS
2 cups water
½ cup quick grits
¾ cup shredded reduced-fat cheddar cheese
1 Tbsp reduced-fat margarine
2 Tbsp chopped green chilies or picante sauce
1 egg, separated
¼ cup fat-free milk

METHOD
1. Preheat oven to 350 degrees.
2. Bring water to boil in heavy saucepan. Stir in grits.
    Return to a boil. Reduce heat, partially cover, and cook
    5 minutes. Stir occasionally.
3. Add cheese, margarine, and chilies. Stir until cheese is
    melted.
4. Beat egg yolk with milk and stir into grits.
5. Whip egg white until stiff and fold into mixture.
6. Pour into 5- by 5-inch casserole dish that has been
    sprayed with nonstick cooking spray and bake for
    1 hour. Let set 5 minutes before cutting.

1 Apple-Raisin Muffin
½ cup bran flakes with
1 cup fat-free milk

33

55g carb

Apple-Raisin Muffins

Yield: 12 muffins / Serving size: 1 muffin

INGREDIENTS

2 cups all-purpose flour
1 Tbsp baking powder
¼ tsp salt
1 tsp cinnamon
3 pkt sugar substitute suitable for baking
1 egg, lightly beaten
3 Tbsp canola oil
½ cup fat-free milk
1 cup unsweetened applesauce
½ cup raisins, soaked in very hot water 15 minutes and
   drained

METHOD

1. Preheat oven to 400 degrees. Prepare 2½-inch muffin
   tins by spraying with cooking spray.
2. Combine dry ingredients in mixing bowl and mix
   thoroughly.
3. Beat egg and whip in oil, milk, and applesauce.
4. Add liquid mixture to dry ingredients and mix until
   flour is moistened. Stir in raisins.
5. Fill muffin tins two-thirds full. Bake for 25 minutes.
   Remove muffins from tin immediately. Store muffins in
   freezer for later use.

34

45g carb

1 serving **Creamed Chipped Beef over Toast**
¾ cup equal parts berries and cubed melon
2 Tbsp granola
1 Tbsp whipped topping

Creamed Chipped Beef over Toast

Yield: 2 servings / Serving size: ½ recipe

INGREDIENTS

2 oz dried beef
2 tsp butter or margarine
1 Tbsp flour
1 cup fat-free or low-fat (1%) milk
2 slices whole-wheat toast

METHOD

1. Pour enough hot water over beef to cover. Soak for 20–30 minutes. Pour off water and slice beef into strips.
2. Melt butter in a small saucepan. Stir in flour with a wooden spoon until well mixed.
3. Add milk a little at a time until all milk is added.
4. Add beef and heat until bubbly.
5. Cut toast in half and pour beef over toast.

35

55g carb

2 **Angel Biscuits**
½ broiled grapefruit
1 cup fat-free milk

Angel Biscuits

Yield: 36 biscuits / Serving size: 1 biscuit

INGREDIENTS
1 pkg. quick-rising yeast
2 Tbsp warm water
3 cups all-purpose white flour
2 cups all-purpose whole-wheat flour
1 tsp baking soda
1 Tbsp baking powder
4 Tbsp sugar
2 tsp salt
1 cup shortening
2 cups reduced-fat buttermilk
Melted butter to brush tops (optional)

METHOD
1. Preheat oven to 400 degrees.
2. Dissolve yeast in lukewarm water.
3. Sift flours, soda, baking powder, sugar, and salt into bowl. Cut in shortening.
4. Add buttermilk, then yeast mixture. Stir until all flour is dampened.
5. Knead on floured board for 1–2 minutes. Roll out to desired thickness and cut with biscuit cutter, or refrigerate dough in an airtight container and use as needed (dough will keep for several days).
6. If desired, brush with melted butter before or after baking on nonstick baking sheet. Bake about 12–15 minutes.

1 serving **Spanish Omelette**
2 slices rye toast with
1 tsp margarine
¾ cup grapefruit sections

Spanish Omelette

Yield: 4 servings / Serving size: ¼ recipe

INGREDIENTS

½ cup chopped green pepper
¼ cup chopped onion
1 Tbsp minced garlic
2 Tbsp water
1 can green chilis, chopped
2 Roma tomatoes, chopped, seeds removed
2 tsp chopped pimiento
6 egg whites
Pinch of saffron
½ cup low-fat cottage cheese (1%)

METHOD

1. In nonstick skillet, sauté green pepper, onion, and garlic in water. Add chilis, tomato, and pimiento and boil off remaining liquid.
2. Combine egg whites and saffron and beat into soft peaks. Fold cottage cheese into egg whites, followed by the contents of the skillet.
3. Return to skillet and fry until eggs are set, turning to avoid scorching. Pour off any water rendered during cooking and serve.

2 4-inch round waffles
2 Tbsp reduced-calorie syrup
1 serving **Grapefruit Grand**
1 cup fat-free or low-fat (1%) milk

37

58g carb

Grapefruit Grand

Yield: 1 serving

INGREDIENTS

½ grapefruit
1 tsp sugar substitute
Dash cinnamon

METHOD

1. Set oven to broil.
2. Top grapefruit with sugar substitute and cinnamon.
3. Broil grapefruit for about 2 minutes.

1 serving **Broccoli Quiche**
½ English muffin with
1 tsp margarine
41g carb   1 cup mixed melon chunks and berries

Broccoli Quiche

Yield: 6 servings / Serving size: ⅙ recipe

INGREDIENTS

1 10-oz pkg. frozen cut broccoli
½ cup chopped green pepper
⅓ cup chopped onion
1 cup shredded Colby cheese
1 cup fat-free milk
½ cup biscuit mix
3 eggs or ¾ cup egg substitute
¼ tsp salt
¼ tsp pepper

METHOD

1. Preheat oven to 375 degrees.
2. Cook broccoli according to package directions; drain.
3. Place broccoli in 9-inch pie plate coated with nonstick cooking spray; sprinkle with green pepper, onion, and cheese. Set aside.
4. Combine remaining ingredients in an electric blender; blend 15 seconds or until smooth. Pour over broccoli mixture.
5. Bake for 25–30 minutes or until set. Let stand 5 minutes before serving.

39

56g carb

2 4-inch **Fluffy High-Fiber, Low-Fat Pancakes** with
½ cup strawberry topping and
1 tsp margarine
2 Tbsp low-fat granola
1 cup fat-free or low-fat (1%) milk

Fluffy High-Fiber, Low-Fat Pancakes

Yield: 8 4-inch pancakes / Serving size: 2 pancakes

INGREDIENTS

1 cup low-fat buttermilk or sour fat-free milk (add 1 Tbsp lemon juice per 1 cup milk)
½ cup quick-cooking oats
⅔ cup miller's bran (unprocessed, uncooked wheat bran)

1 egg
¼ cup whole-wheat flour
½ tsp sugar
¼ tsp salt
¾ tsp baking soda
1 cup strawberries, fresh or frozen, no sugar added
1 tsp apple juice concentrate

METHOD

1. Combine buttermilk, oats, and bran in large mixing bowl. Let stand 5 minutes. Add egg and beat until blended.
2. Mix flour, sugar, salt, and baking soda until blended.
3. Add to bran mixture and blend until flour is moistened.
4. Pour ¼ cup batter in hot nonstick frying pan. Cook about 3 minutes or until bubbles form and edge of pancake is dry. Turn and cook 2 minutes longer.
5. Top with ½ cup strawberry topping. To make strawberry topping, place 1 cup strawberries and 1 tsp apple juice concentrate in blender. Blend until smooth.

40

46g carb

1 slice **Tofu Garden Quiche**
2 slices whole-wheat toast
1 Tbsp reduced-fat margarine
½ cup mixed fresh fruit

Tofu Garden Quiche

Yield: 8 slices / Serving size: 1 slice

INGREDIENTS

2 tsp canola oil
½ medium onion, finely
  chopped
2 cups cooked chopped
  vegetables (use a colorful
  assortment, such as red
  and green peppers and
  yellow squash)
2 eggs or ½ cup egg
  substitute

1 lb tofu, drained, divided in
  two
1 Tbsp lemon juice
1 tsp dried oregano
1 tsp dried dill
½ tsp dried thyme
¼ tsp salt
⅛ tsp garlic powder
⅛ tsp ground nutmeg
¼ cup Parmesan cheese

METHOD

1. Preheat oven to 325 degrees. Heat oil in a large skillet.
   Add onion and cook until onion is soft, about 5
   minutes.
2. Add cooked vegetables and mix. Remove from heat and
   set aside.
3. Put eggs and half of the tofu into a blender and blend
   until smooth and creamy. Add remaining ingredients—
   except vegetable mixture and Parmesan cheese—and
   blend until smooth. Mix vegetables into tofu mixture.
4. Pour the tofu mixture into a large quiche dish or pie pan.
5. Sprinkle with Parmesan cheese.
6. Bake for 50–60 minutes or until knife comes out clean.

1 Peanut Butter and Jelly Muffin
1 cup fat-free fruit-flavored yogurt
½ grapefruit

41

63g carb

Peanut Butter and Jelly Muffins

Yield: 12 muffins / Serving size: 1 muffin

INGREDIENTS

2 cups flour
3 Tbsp sugar
1 Tbsp baking powder
¾ cup creamy peanut butter
1 egg
1 cup low-fat (1%) milk
⅓ cup 100% fruit spread (raspberry or strawberry)

METHOD

1. Preheat oven to 350 degrees.
2. Spray muffin tin with vegetable spray or line with baking cups.
3. In a large bowl, mix flour, sugar, and baking powder.
4. In another bowl, beat peanut butter and egg until smooth. Add milk a little at a time, stirring after each addition.
5. Pour peanut butter mixture over dry ingredients; fold in with a rubber spatula just until dry ingredients are moistened. Batter will be stiff.
6. Spoon 2 scant tablespoons of batter into each muffin cup and smooth the surface out to the top edge of the cup. Then top each muffin with a heaping teaspoon of fruit spread; cover with 2 more tablespoons of batter.
7. Bake 20–25 minutes or until lightly browned.

2 Iowa Corn Pancakes with
2 Tbsp sugar-free syrup and
1 Tbsp reduced-fat margarine
1 cup fat-free milk

57g carb

Iowa Corn Pancakes

Yield: 8 pancakes / Serving size: 1 pancake

INGREDIENTS

1 cup sour low-fat (1%) milk (add 1 Tbsp white vinegar per
    1 cup milk)
½ cup quick-cooking oats
1 cup whole-kernel corn (leftovers or canned can be used)
¼ cup all-purpose flour
¼ cup whole-wheat flour
¼ tsp salt
¾ tsp baking soda
¼ cup egg substitute

METHOD

1. Combine milk, oats, and corn in a large mixing bowl
   and let stand for 8 minutes.
2. Mix flours, salt, and baking soda in a small bowl and set
   aside.
3. Add egg substitute to milk mixture and beat until
   blended.
4. Add dry ingredients to wet ingredients and stir until just
   mixed.
5. Pour slightly less than ⅓ cup batter on a hot griddle that
   has been sprayed with nonstick cooking spray.
6. Cook until bubbles form on edges and edges start to dry.
7. Turn and cook 2–3 more minutes.

2 Sweet Potato–Raisin Cookies
1 small banana
1 cup fat-free or low-fat (1%) milk

59g carb

Sweet Potato–Raisin Cookies

Yield 24 cookies / Serving size: 2 cookies

INGREDIENTS

1 cup raisins
¼ cup butter or margarine
1 cup sweet potatoes,
  cooked and mashed
1 egg
1 tsp vanilla
2 cups whole-wheat flour
¼ tsp allspice

½ tsp salt
½ tsp nutmeg
½ tsp baking soda
1 tsp baking powder
1 tsp cinnamon
¼ cup walnuts, chopped
½ cup unprocessed bran
  flakes

METHOD

1. Preheat oven to 350 degrees. Soak raisins in hot water to cover for 5 minutes, then drain.
2. Cream margarine, then add sweet potatoes, egg, and vanilla; beat until creamy.
3. Mix flour, allspice, salt, nutmeg, baking soda, baking powder, and cinnamon. Add to creamed mixture and mix well.
4. Add raisins, nuts, and bran.
5. Drop onto cookie sheet that has been sprayed with nonstick cooking spray.
6. Bake for 12 minutes or until done.

44

58g carb

1 serving **Baked Rice Pudding**
3 stewed prunes
2 Tbsp roasted almonds
1 cup fat-free or low-fat (1%) milk

Baked Rice Pudding

Yield: 4 servings / Serving size: ¼ recipe

INGREDIENTS

1 cup fat-free milk
2 eggs, slightly beaten
1 Tbsp sugar
⅛ tsp salt
1 tsp vanilla
2 cups cooked rice (or other whole grain)
⅛ tsp grated nutmeg (optional)
Sugar substitute to taste (optional)

METHOD

1. Preheat oven to 325 degrees.
2. Heat milk in the top of a double boiler over simmering water until surface begins to wrinkle.
3. Blend together eggs, sugar, salt, and vanilla. Add hot milk gradually, stirring to mix well.
4. Add rice. Pour into four 6-oz individual custard cups. Sprinkle surface lightly with nutmeg.
5. Set cups in a deep pan; pour hot water around cups to within ½ inch of tops of cups.
6. Bake 50–60 minutes or until toothpick comes out clean.
7. Remove cups from pan. Chill for several hours before serving.
8. Sprinkle with sugar substitute, if desired.

45

50g carb

1 serving **Low Country Grits and Sausage**
¾ cup fresh citrus sections

Low Country Grits and Sausage

Yield: 2 servings / Serving size: ½ recipe

INGREDIENTS

½ cup uncooked yellow or white grits (stone ground are best)
2 oz turkey sausage, cooked and crumbled
2 eggs, beaten
½ cup fat-free milk
½ tsp thyme
⅛ tsp garlic salt (optional)

METHOD

1. Cook grits according to package directions.
2. Combine sausage, eggs, milk, thyme, and garlic salt in medium bowl. Add a small amount of hot grits and mix well. Add mixture to rest of grits.
3. Mix well and pour into a loaf pan that has been coated with nonstick cooking spray. Cover and refrigerate overnight.
4. Next morning, remove from refrigerator and let stand 15 minutes before baking.
5. Preheat oven to 350 degrees. Bake for 45 minutes or until done.

1 slice **Johnnycake** with
1½ tsp reduced-fat margarine
⅔ cup raspberries with
Sugar substitute (optional)
2 oz turkey ham
4 oz orange juice

46

45g carb

Johnnycake

Yield: 1 loaf of 12 slices / Serving size: 1 slice

INGREDIENTS
2 cups cornmeal
1½ tsp salt
1 tsp baking soda
2 Tbsp sugar
2 cups buttermilk
½ cup egg substitute
2 Tbsp canola oil

METHOD
1. Preheat oven to 400 degrees.
2. Mix dry ingredients together.
3. Add buttermilk, egg substitute, and oil.
4. Mix well. Pour into 8- by 10-inch loaf pan coated with nonstick cooking spray.
5. Bake for 30 minutes.

1 serving **Granola Pancakes**
½ Tbsp reduced-calorie margarine
2 Tbsp apple butter or ½ cup unsweetened
applesauce

47

62g carb

Granola Pancakes

Yield: About 18 4-inch pancakes / Serving size: 3 pancakes

INGREDIENTS
2 eggs or 1 egg plus 2 egg whites
2 cups fat-free milk
2 Tbsp molasses
2 cups whole-wheat flour
½ cup low-fat granola
2 tsp baking powder

METHOD
1. Beat eggs in a large cup or bowl; add milk and molasses and stir.
2. Combine flour, granola, and baking powder and add to liquid mixture, mixing lightly with a fork.
3. Coat skillet with nonstick cooking spray and heat over medium heat.
4. Drop pancake batter, using about ¼ cup per pancake, onto skillet. Turn pancakes once. Cook until golden brown on both sides.

1 **Atomic Muffin**
½ cups cooked grits
1 cup cubed honeydew melon

Atomic Muffins

Yield: 24 muffins / Serving size: 1 muffin

INGREDIENTS

½ cup canola or safflower oil
¼ cup brown sugar
2 Tbsp. molasses
2 eggs
¾ cup wheat germ
1 cup whole-wheat flour
¼ cup soy flour
½ cup fat-free dry milk
½ cup ground sesame seeds
½ cup chopped sunflower seeds
1½ cups low-fat milk or vanilla-flavored soy milk
2 tsp. baking powder
1 cup raisins
1 cup chopped nuts
⅛ cup rolled oats

METHOD

1. Preheat oven to 375 degrees. Mix the first 4 ingredients in a large mixing bowl. Add remaining ingredients and mix well.
2. Put paper cups in muffin tins or spray tins with nonstick cooking spray. Fill cups ⅔ full with batter. Bake 18 minutes.

49

1 serving **Oatmeal-Wheatena Porridge with Banana and Walnuts**
½ cup fat-free milk

56g carb

Oatmeal-Wheatena Porridge with Banana and Walnuts

Yield: 1 serving

INGREDIENTS
1 cup water
3 Tbsp Wheatena
¼ cup quick-cooking oats
½ small banana, mashed
1 tsp sugar substitute
1 tsp vanilla
1 Tbsp chopped walnuts

METHOD
1. Add Wheatena to boiling water. Cook 2-3 minutes over moderate heat, then add oats.
2. Cook to desired consistency. Mix in the mashed banana, sugar substitute, and vanilla.
3. Pour into bowl and top with chopped walnuts.

50

60g carb

2 **Whole-Wheat Currant Scones**
1 cup fat-free artificially sweetened vanilla
yogurt

Whole-Wheat Currant Scones

Yield: 16 scones / Serving size: 2 scones

INGREDIENTS

1 cup whole-wheat pastry
flour
1 cup all-purpose white flour
1 cup quick-cooking oats
½ cup oat bran
2 Tbsp baking powder
¼ tsp salt
¼ tsp cream of tartar

4 Tbsp reduced-fat
margarine
½ cup currants
⅔ cup fat-free plain yogurt
1 Tbsp vanilla
¼ cup orange juice
¼ cup sugar
2 eggs

METHOD

1. Preheat oven to 425 degrees.
2. Mix flours, oats, oat bran, baking powder, salt, and cream
   of tartar in a bowl.
3. Cut in margarine until mixture is mealy. Add currants
   and mix until coated with flour.
4. In a small bowl, mix together yogurt, vanilla, orange
   juice, sugar, and eggs and add to dry ingredients, mixing
   just until a ball of dough forms. If mixture is too dry, add
   1–2 Tbsp more yogurt.
5. Knead dough on floured pastry cloth about 10 times.
   Divide dough in half, and form two circles of dough about
   ½ inch thick.
6. Transfer to baking sheet coated with nonstick cooking
   spray, and cut each circle into 8 pie-shaped wedges.
7. Bake for 12–15 minutes.

Lunch

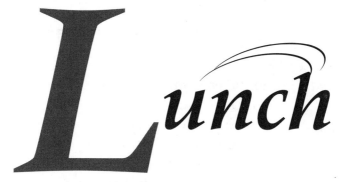

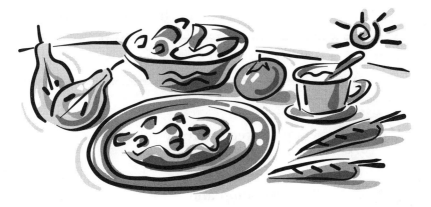

Each lunch in this section has about 450 calories and includes
2–3 starch servings
1–2 meat or meat substitute
    servings
0–2 vegetable servings
1 fruit serving
1 fat serving

Average Fat: 15 grams

Average Carbohydrate: 50 grams

Average Protein: 22 grams

Some menus have 1 fat-free milk serving instead of 1 meat or 1 starch serving. Or 1 starch serving instead of the fruit serving.

No-Fuss Noons

52g carb

1 cup vegetable soup
6 saltine crackers
½ Chicken Sandwich:
    1 slice whole-wheat bread
    2 oz chicken breast
    1 tsp mayonnaise
    Lettuce, tomato, and mustard, as desired
1 orange or ⅓ cup fat-free frozen yogurt

57g carb

3 oz lean ham
⅓ cup cooked white or yellow rice
½ cup black beans with
1 tsp olive oil and
Chopped onion and
Vinegar to taste
½ cup turnip greens with
Hot pepper sauce to taste
2 figs

Chef's Salad:
2 cups lettuce
Chopped raw vegetables
1 oz ham, turkey, or chicken
1 oz cheese
2 tomato wedges
2 Tbsp reduced-fat salad dressing
2 RyKrisp crackers
1¼ cups strawberries
3 oz frozen low-fat yogurt

57g carb

Reuben Sandwich:
2 slices toasted rye bread
1 oz cooked corned beef, sliced
¾ oz part-skim mozzarella cheese, sliced
1 Tbsp Thousand Island salad dressing
¼ cup sauerkraut, rinsed and drained
½ cup pears canned in juice

50g carb

Make sandwich, wrap in paper towel, and microwave for 15 seconds or until heated.

1 10¾-oz can chunky beef and vegetable
    soup
1 slice whole-wheat toast with
1 oz melted Monterey Jack cheese
17 grapes

50g carb

Macaroni Salad:
1 cup cooked macaroni, drained and chilled
2 oz part-skim mozzarella cheese cubes
2 Tbsp chopped green pepper
2 Tbsp chopped carrots
2 Tbsp chopped onions
1 Tbsp reduced-fat mayonnaise
1 Tbsp fat-free plain yogurt
1 kiwi fruit

6
61g carb

1 Vegetable-Topped Potato:
6-oz baking potato, microwaved, topped with
¼ cup low-fat cottage cheese
2 Tbsp shredded cheddar cheese
¼ cup broccoli florets
¼ cup chopped tomato
¼ cup chopped green onions
¼ cup sliced mushrooms
1 small apple

7
71g carb

Stouffer's Lean Cuisine Lasagna with Meat
  Sauce
Tossed salad
63g carb 2 Tbsp reduced-fat salad dressing
1 small banana

Pasta Salad:
  1 cup pasta, cooked
  ¼ cup water-packed canned tuna,
    drained
62g carb 1 oz shredded cheddar cheese
  1 cup mixture of broccoli, cucumber, and
    green, red, or yellow peppers
  2 Tbsp reduced-fat salad dressing
  1 small tomato, cut into wedges
1 small nectarine

1 energy or cereal bar (Balance Bar)
3 cups air-popped (fat-free) popcorn
1 Tbsp reduced-fat margarine
1 cup carrot sticks
70g carb 4 dried apple rings

Chicken pita pocket sandwich:
1 6-inch pita bread
2 oz chopped cooked chicken breast
58g carb   ¼ cup shredded lettuce
¼ cup green bell pepper strips
¼ cup sliced mushrooms
¼ cup chopped tomato
2 Tbsp reduced-fat salad dressing
¾ cup Mandarin oranges

1 piece Boston Market turkey breast
1 single serving Boston Market corn
1 single serving Boston Market coleslaw
47g carb   1 small apple

Quesadillas:
  2 6-inch flour tortillas
  2 oz shredded reduced-fat cheddar cheese
  ¼ cup salsa
1 cup carrot sticks

13

52g carb

Coat skillet with cooking spray, then heat. Put 1 tortilla in pan and sprinkle with cheese. Cover with second tortilla. Brown on both sides. Dip in salsa.

14

78g carb

½ cup canned kidney beans, rinsed and
  drained, heated with
Finely diced onion, garlic, and green pepper
  to taste
⅓ cup tomato sauce with
Cajun seasoning to taste over
⅔ cup cooked brown rice
Tossed green salad with
1 Tbsp reduced-fat Ranch dressing
2 Tbsp raisins

LUNCH

15

47g carb

1 Salmon Pita Pocket Sandwich:
    1 6-inch whole-wheat pita pocket
    ½ cup canned salmon, drained, with
    1 Tbsp reduced-fat mayonnaise
    ½ cup shredded lettuce
    2 tomato slices
1¼ cups watermelon cubes

16

57g carb

Stuffed Baked Potato:
    1 medium baked potato topped with
    2 oz shredded cheddar cheese and
    ¼ cup chopped cooked broccoli
1 nectarine

17

52g carb

4 RyKrisp crackers
Shrimp Salad:
   4 oz shrimp
   Bed of lettuce and fresh raw vegetables,
     as desired
   1 chopped tomato
   $\frac{1}{8}$ avocado with
   2 Tbsp **French Dressing**
$\frac{1}{2}$ cup grapefruit sections

French Dressing

Yield: 6 servings / Serving size: 2 Tbsp

INGREDIENTS

$\frac{1}{2}$ cup tomato juice
2 Tbsp lemon juice or vinegar
1 Tbsp finely chopped onion
1 Tbsp finely chopped green pepper
1 tsp minced garlic
$\frac{1}{4}$ tsp salt
$\frac{1}{8}$ tsp black pepper

METHOD

Combine all ingredients in a jar. Cover and shake well before using.

18

54g carb

1 slice **Whole-Wheat Pizza**
Tossed salad with
1 Tbsp Italian dressing
1 cup honeydew melon cubes

Whole-Wheat Pizza

Yield: 8 servings / Serving size: 1 slice

LUNCH

INGREDIENTS

1 cup warm water
(110–115 degrees)
1 pkg. (or 1 Tbsp) active dry
yeast or 1 cake yeast
1 Tbsp honey
2 cups whole-wheat flour
½ tsp salt
1 Tbsp canola oil
4 oz shredded reduced-fat
cheddar cheese
Fresh ground pepper

½ cup unbleached white
flour
½ cup water (if necessary)
¼ tsp garlic powder
1 Tbsp cornmeal
½ cup tomato or pizza sauce
1 Tbsp oregano
1 cup chopped broccoli
1 cup sliced mushrooms
½ cup shredded part-skim
mozzarella cheese

METHOD

1. Combine water, yeast, honey, and 1 cup of whole-wheat
   flour in a large bowl. Beat 5 minutes until mixture is
   smooth. Let rise in a warm place for 15 minutes.
2. Add salt, oil, cheddar cheese, pepper, white flour, water (if
   needed), garlic powder, and remaining whole-wheat flour
   to the dough.
3. Mix well and let the dough rest for 5 minutes.
4. Preheat oven to 400 degrees. Pat out dough onto a
   baking sheet dusted with cornmeal, building up sides to
   form a crust.
5. Top with the pizza sauce, oregano, vegetables, and
   mozzarella. Bake for 15–20 minutes.

19

60g carb

1 cup **Noodle Supreme Salad**
6 Triscuits
1 tsp margarine
1 apple

Noodle Supreme Salad

Yield: 2 servings / Serving size: 1 cup

INGREDIENTS

3 cups water
2 oz wide noodles
¼ cup frozen peas
3 Tbsp low-fat cream of mushroom soup
2 oz water-packed canned tuna, drained
2 Tbsp shredded red cabbage
¼ cup diced tomatoes
2 Romaine lettuce leaves
2 Tbsp chopped green onion

METHOD

1. Bring water to a boil. Add noodles and peas. Cook uncovered 5 minutes. Drain.
2. Combine noodles, peas, soup, and tuna. Mix lightly. Cool.
3. Add red cabbage and tomatoes.
4. Serve on lettuce leaves and garnish with chopped green onion.

LUNCH

1 cup **Black Bean Soup**
6 saltine crackers
Tossed salad with
72g carb 2 Tbsp reduced-fat salad dressing
½ cup unsweetened canned fruit cocktail

20

Black Bean Soup

Yield: 4 servings / Serving size: 1 cup

LUNCH

INGREDIENTS

½ lb dried black beans
1 qt water
1 Tbsp olive oil
1 cup chopped onions
½ cup chopped green bell
   pepper

1 Tbsp minced garlic
½ tsp cumin
½ tsp oregano
¼ tsp dry mustard
1 Tbsp lemon juice
2 Tbsp minced green onion

METHOD

1. Presoak beans in water overnight or use quick-cook method on package.
2. After soaking beans, drain, refill water, and bring to a boil; cover and simmer on low heat for 2 hours.
3. Heat oil, add onions, and sauté about 5 minutes. Add green pepper and sauté until onions are tender.
4. Stir in remaining ingredients. Add about ¾ cup hot bean liquid, cover, and simmer 10 minutes.
5. Add onion seasoning mixture to beans and continue to cook 1 hour, stirring occasionally.
6. To serve, top with green onion.

21	1 **Sloppy Joe** on
	Hamburger bun
	Raw carrot and celery sticks
66g carb	1 apple
	5 vanilla wafers

Sloppy Joes

Yield: 6 servings / Serving size: ½ cup

INGREDIENTS

1 lb lean ground beef or ground turkey breast
½ cup chopped onion
½ cup chopped celery
1 8-oz can tomato sauce
¼ tsp cumin
½ tsp onion powder
½ Tbsp Worcestershire sauce
Dash pepper
6 hamburger buns (preferably whole grain)

METHOD

1. Sauté ground beef, onion, and celery. Drain excess fat.
2. Add remaining ingredients. Simmer 10 minutes.
3. Spoon onto hamburger buns, allowing about ½ cup per bun.

LUNCH

1 cup chicken noodle soup
1 **English Muffin Pizza Melt**
Tossed salad with
2 Tbsp reduced-fat salad dressing
1 pear

22

66g carb

English Muffin Pizza Melt

Yield: 6 servings / Serving size: ½ muffin

INGREDIENTS

1 lb lean ground beef
¼ cup chopped onion
1 8-oz can pizza sauce
2 tsp minced fresh parsley
½ tsp basil
¼ tsp garlic powder
2 Tbsp shredded part-skim mozzarella cheese
3 English muffins, split

METHOD

1. Preheat oven to 350 degrees.
2. Cook beef and onion until meat is no longer pink. Drain fat. Stir in pizza sauce and seasonings and simmer 2 minutes.
3. If desired, toast muffins. Top each muffin with ⅙ cup beef mixture. Top with 1 tsp cheese.
4. Bake for 10–15 minutes or until heated thoroughly and cheese is melted.

LUNCH

1 Tortilla Ranch Style
1 small nectarine

23

58g carb

Tortilla Ranch Style

Yield: 1 serving

INGREDIENTS

1 cup assorted vegetables (carrots, celery, zucchini, green
  onions, spinach, sweet red peppers, and/or lettuce),
  thinly shredded
1 large flour tortilla
2 Tbsp reduced-fat Ranch dressing
1 oz Swiss cheese
1 oz sliced turkey

METHOD

1. Layer vegetables on tortilla.
2. Sprinkle dressing over vegetables.
3. Add Swiss cheese and turkey. Roll up. Eat cold or
   microwave briefly.

LUNCH

1 Submarine Sandwich
3 mixed nuts
½ large pear

51g carb

Submarine Sandwich

Yield: 4 sandwiches / Serving size: 1 sandwich

INGREDIENTS
½ loaf (½ lb) French bread
½ Tbsp mustard, or to taste
2 oz part-skim mozzarella cheese, sliced
¼ lb turkey, sliced
1 cup shredded lettuce
1 medium tomato, thinly sliced
½ medium onion, thinly sliced
2 oz cooked smoked ham, thinly sliced
½ medium green pepper, thinly sliced
2 Tbsp reduced-fat Italian dressing

METHOD
1. Cut bread into halves horizontally. Spread bottom half with mustard.
2. Layer cheese, turkey, lettuce, tomatoes, onion, ham, and green pepper on top. Drizzle with dressing; top with remaining bread half. Secure loaf with long toothpicks. To serve, cut into 4 pieces.

25

60g carb

1 cup **Minestrone**
2 RyKrisp crackers
2 oz fat-free mozzarella cheese
1 ¼ cups fresh strawberries

Minestrone

Yield: 5 servings / Serving size: 1 cup

INGREDIENTS

½ cup chopped onion
2 cloves garlic, minced
1 ½ tsp olive oil
1 qt low-sodium, low-fat
   beef or chicken broth
½ cup sliced zucchini
⅓ cup chopped carrot
1 rib celery, chopped
1 14-oz can Italian plum
   tomatoes

1 15-oz can cannellini or
   navy beans, rinsed and
   drained
½ cup shredded cabbage
½ cup peeled, cubed potato
1 tsp basil
Fresh ground pepper
1 Tbsp tomato paste
½ 10-oz pkg. frozen Italian-
   style green beans
¼ cup elbow macaroni
¼ cup Parmesan cheese

METHOD

1. In large stock pot, sauté onion and garlic in olive oil
   until soft but not brown (about 10 minutes). Add
   remaining ingredients, except Italian green beans, pasta,
   and Parmesan cheese.
2. Bring to a boil, cover, reduce heat, and simmer for 1 hour.
3. Stir in beans, pasta, and half the Parmesan cheese.
   Simmer for an additional 15 minutes.
4. Season to taste. Serve hot or at room temperature with
   remaining Parmesan cheese.

LUNCH

1 serving **Spicy Black-Eyed Peas**
2 oz hamburger patty
Tossed salad with
2 Tbsp reduced-fat salad dressing and
1 Tbsp shredded cheddar cheese
1 small orange

52g carb

Spicy Black-Eyed Peas

Yield: 4 servings / Serving size: 1¼ cups

INGREDIENTS

½ cup chopped onion
½ cup chopped green pepper
1 16-oz can black-eyed peas, undrained
1 16-oz can stewed tomatoes, undrained
1 tsp dry mustard
½ tsp chili powder
⅛ tsp red pepper
½ tsp pepper
1 Tbsp lite soy sauce
1 tsp liquid smoke
1 Tbsp minced fresh parsley

METHOD

1. Coat a large nonstick skillet with nonstick cooking spray; place over medium heat until hot.
2. Add onion and green pepper; sauté until vegetables are tender-crisp.
3. Add remaining ingredients except parsley; bring to a boil. Reduce heat; simmer 20 minutes, stirring often. Transfer to a serving dish. Sprinkle with parsley.

LUNCH

1 serving **Crunchy Tuna Cheese Melt**
1 cup vegetable soup
5 peanuts
51g carb   4 canned apricot halves, unsweetened

Crunchy Tuna Cheese Melt

Yield: 1 serving / Serving size: 2 slices

INGREDIENTS

½ cup water-packed canned tuna, drained
2 Tbsp fat-free plain yogurt
4 water chestnuts, sliced
2 Tbsp chopped onion
2 Tbsp chopped celery
2 slices whole-wheat bread, toasted
¼ cup shredded Monterey Jack cheese
2 green pepper rings

METHOD

1. Set oven to broil.
2. In small bowl, combine tuna, yogurt, water chestnuts, onions, and celery.
3. Spread on toasted bread. Top with shredded cheese and broil until cheese melts. Garnish each slice with a green pepper ring.

LUNCH

1 serving Fast Corn Chowder
½ cup cottage cheese on lettuce leaf
1 cup sliced cucumber
1 Tbsp reduced-fat salad dressing
1 cup melon balls

28

58g carb

Fast Corn Chowder

Yield: 4 servings / Serving size: 1 cup

INGREDIENTS

1 17-oz can cream-style corn
1 12-oz can whole kernel corn with sweet peppers, undrained
1 12-oz can or 1½ cups evaporated fat-free milk
1 tsp dried minced onion
Dash pepper
1 Tbsp margarine

METHOD

1. In a medium saucepan, combine all ingredients except margarine.
2. Bring to a boil, stirring constantly. Add margarine. Serve.

Veggie Pizza
1 cup cantaloupe cubes
½ cup fat-free artificially sweetened ice cream

29

74g carb

Veggie Pizza

Yield: 2 servings / Serving size: 1 piece

INGREDIENTS
1 5-oz Boboli pizza crust
⅔ cup pizza sauce
½ tsp garlic powder
1 tsp oregano
½ cup shredded part-skim mozzarella cheese
2 Tbsp chopped onion
2 Tbsp chopped bell pepper
2 Tbsp sliced mushrooms

METHOD
1. Preheat oven to 450 degrees.
2. Place crust on rack on top of cookie sheet. Spread sauce on top.
3. Sprinkle remaining ingredients over sauce and bake for 8–10 minutes.

L U N C H

1 serving **Light Spinach Salad**
1 slice French bread
1 tsp margarine

48g carb

Light Spinach Salad

Yield: 2 servings / Serving size: ½ recipe

INGREDIENTS
4 cups torn fresh spinach
4 oz cooked boneless skinless chicken breast, cubed
1 medium orange, peeled, seeded, and sectioned
½ cup sliced mushrooms
1 small onion, sliced
2 oz cheddar cheese, cubed or in strips
2 Tbsp reduced-fat salad dressing

METHOD
1. Combine all ingredients except cheese and dressing in a large bowl; chill.
2. Before serving, add cheese and toss with dressing.

1 serving **Gazpacho**
2 slices whole-wheat bread
½ cup egg salad made with
1 Tbsp reduced-fat mayonnaise
1 small nectarine

31

58g carb

Gazpacho

Yield: 4 servings / Serving size: 1 cup

INGREDIENTS
4 medium tomatoes, quartered
1 small cucumber, peeled and sliced
¼ cup sliced onion
1 medium carrot, finely diced
2 stalks celery, quartered
½ green pepper, sliced
1 clove garlic, minced
1 tsp salt
¼ tsp pepper
2 Tbsp olive oil
3 Tbsp wine vinegar
⅔ cup V-8 juice

METHOD
1. Core and remove seeds from 1 tomato. Chop finely; set aside.
2. Combine all other ingredients in blender. Blend only a few seconds. Mixture should not be smooth.
3. Add chopped tomato. Chill.
4. Serve in chilled bowls with an ice cube in each serving.

LUNCH

1 Broiled Open-Faced Vegetarian Sandwich
1 small banana

76g carb

Broiled Open-Faced Vegetarian Sandwich

Yield: 1 serving

INGREDIENTS
2 slices Italian bread, 1 inch thick
2 tsp reduced-fat margarine
Tomato slices
Zucchini slices
Onion slices
Green pepper slices
Garlic powder
Basil
Pepper
2 oz shredded part-skim mozzarella cheese

METHOD
1. Spread bread with 1 tsp margarine on each piece.
2. Top with tomato, zucchini, onion, and green pepper slices.
3. Sprinkle with garlic powder, basil, and pepper; top with cheese.
4. Broil until browned on edges and cheese is melted.

33

62g carb

1 slice cold **Spicy Turkey Loaf**
2 slices reduced-calorie bread (40 calories each)
Lettuce and tomato slice or ketchup, as desired
½ mango or 12 cherries

Spicy Turkey Loaf

Yield: 8 servings / Serving size: 1 slice

INGREDIENTS

1½ lb lean ground turkey
¾ cup fat-free evaporated milk
¼ cup finely chopped onion
¾ cup bread crumbs
4 Tbsp chili sauce
½ tsp ground ginger
½ tsp crushed fresh garlic clove
A few parsley or cilantro leaves, chopped

METHOD

1. Preheat oven to 350 degrees.
2. Mix all ingredients together. Press into an ungreased loaf pan.
3. Bake 45 minutes or until toothpick comes out clean. Cool about 5 minutes, then cut into 8 slices.

2 Pizza Muffins
4 Tbsp Parmesan cheese
Tossed salad with
2 Tbsp reduced-fat dressing
1 apple

34

57g carb

Pizza Muffins

Yield: 12 muffins / Serving size: 2 muffins

INGREDIENTS

1 egg
½ cup tomato sauce
1 cup low-fat buttermilk or
   low-fat plain yogurt
1 tsp oregano
¼ tsp garlic powder
¼ tsp freshly ground pepper

½ cup shredded part-skim
   mozzarella cheese, divided
1½ cups whole-wheat flour
3 Tbsp wheat germ
2 tsp baking powder
1 tsp baking soda
2 sliced Roma tomatoes
1 Tbsp sesame seeds

METHOD

1. Preheat oven to 400 degrees. Spray muffin tin with cooking spray or line with baking cups.
2. Blend egg, tomato sauce, and buttermilk with a mixer or food processor. Add spices. Add ¼ cup cheese, reserving remainder for topping.
3. In another bowl, mix flour, wheat germ, baking powder, and baking soda.
4. Combine the two mixtures until flour is no longer visible. Spoon batter into muffin tin, filling each well about two-thirds full. Top each muffin with a slice of tomato and some cheese; sprinkle with sesame seeds.
5. Bake 20–25 minutes.

LUNCH

1 serving **Fiesta Rice**
1 oz shredded cheddar cheese
½ cup green beans
3 medium prunes
Tossed salad
1 Tbsp creamy Ranch dressing

Fiesta Rice

Yield: 4 servings / Serving size: 1 cup

INGREDIENTS

1 cup low-fat shredded cheddar cheese or Farmer's cheese, divided
2½ cups cooked brown rice
¾ cup low-fat cottage cheese (1%)
1 2-oz jar pimientos, drained and chopped
½ cup fat-free milk
1 large tomato, peeled and diced
Dash paprika

METHOD

1. Preheat oven to 350 degrees.
2. Combine ½ cup of cheddar cheese and all other ingredients except paprika. Stir until well mixed.
3. Spray casserole with nonstick cooking spray.
4. Pour in mixture; top with remaining cheddar cheese and sprinkle well with paprika.
5. Bake 25–30 minutes.

LUNCH

1 serving **Turkey-Squash Casserole**
¾ cup mixed citrus fruit sections
Tossed salad
½ Tbsp reduced-fat salad dressing

36

63g carb

Turkey-Squash Casserole

Yield: 6 servings / Serving size: ⅙ recipe

INGREDIENTS

2 Tbsp margarine
1 medium onion, chopped
1½ lb yellow squash, sliced
1 cup shredded carrots
3 cups Pepperidge Farm stuffing mix
1 cup fat-free sour cream
1 egg
1 cup fat-free reduced-sodium chicken broth or enough
   to moisten
12 oz skinless turkey breast, cubed

METHOD

1. Preheat oven to 375 degrees.
2. Sauté onion in margarine. Mix with remaining
   ingredients.
4. Pour into 2-qt baking dish coated with nonstick cooking
   spray.
5. Bake 30–40 minutes or until bubbly.

1 serving **Pan-Broiled Shrimp**
1 medium tomato, sliced
1 cup cooked grits
¾ cup fresh pineapple

Pan-Broiled Shrimp

Yield: 2 servings / Serving size: ½ recipe

INGREDIENTS

1 tsp margarine
⅓ medium sweet onion, sliced
⅓ lb shrimp, peeled and deveined
Lemon juice, salt, and pepper to taste

METHOD

1. Heat margarine in medium saucepan. Sauté onion until translucent.
2. Add shrimp. Sauté until pink, about 3–5 minutes.
3. Add lemon juice, salt, and pepper.

LUNCH

	1 cup **Spanish Garbanzo Beans**
38	½ cup sliced cucumbers in red wine vinegar
	½ cup grapes
60g carb	

Spanish Garbanzo Beans

Yield: 2 servings / Serving size: 1 cup

INGREDIENTS

½ cup chopped onions
1 medium green pepper, chopped
2 Tbsp olive oil
8 oz tomato sauce
1¼ cups garbanzo beans, rinsed and drained

METHOD

1. Sauté onions and pepper in oil. Add tomato sauce. Cook over medium heat for 5 minutes.
2. Add garbanzo beans. Cook over low heat for 15 minutes.

39

53g carb

1 serving **Schinkennudelin**
1 slice bread
1 cup sliced cucumbers
1 Tbsp reduced-fat Cucumber Ranch dressing
17 grapes

Schinkennudelin

Yield: 1 serving

INGREDIENTS

1 oz low-fat ham, cubed
1 Tbsp reduced-calorie margarine
½ cup cooked noodles
1 egg, beaten

METHOD

1. Brown ham cubes in margarine.
2. Add noodles and brown.
3. Add beaten egg and cook, turning in sections, until egg is done.

LUNCH

Lentil-Veggie Soup

Yield: 4 servings / Serving size: 1½ cups

INGREDIENTS

1 Tbsp canola oil
1 large onion, diced
1 clove garlic, minced
2 large carrots, diced
¾ cup celery, chopped
1 10-oz pkg. frozen spinach, thawed
6 oz turkey ham, cubed
Italian seasoning to taste
2 cups dried lentils, picked over and rinsed

METHOD

1. Heat oil in a large stock pot and sauté onion, garlic, and carrots 2–3 minutes.
2. Add celery, spinach, ham, and seasoning and sauté 3–4 minutes.
3. Add lentils and water to cover by 3 inches. Bring to boil, then reduce heat, cover, and simmer 60 minutes.

41	1 serving **Seven-Layer Salad**
	3 pieces Wasa Crisp Bread
56g carb	1 small Granny Smith apple

Seven-Layer Salad

Yield: 2 servings / Serving size: ½ recipe

INGREDIENTS

3 cups torn iceberg lettuce
1 cup frozen green peas, thawed
¼ cup chopped onions
½ cup chopped celery
¼ cup chopped green pepper
¼ cup fat-free plain yogurt
2 Tbsp reduced-fat mayonnaise
2 oz shredded reduced-fat cheddar cheese
2 slices bacon, cooked crisp, drained, and crumbled
2 hard-boiled eggs, sliced

METHOD

1. In a medium casserole dish, layer lettuce and other vegetables.
2. Mix together yogurt and mayonnaise and spread on the top layer. Top with cheese, bacon, and eggs.
3. Cover with plastic wrap and refrigerate 8 hours or more.

1 serving **Caesar Salad**
2 small crisp bread sticks
1 cup frozen melon balls (half cantaloupe, half honeydew)

42

47g carb

Caesar Salad

Yield: 2 servings / Serving size: ½ recipe

INGREDIENTS

1 medium head romaine lettuce
Dressing:
   1 clove garlic, crushed
   ½ tsp black pepper
   2 oz smoked anchovies, drained and patted dry
   1 egg yolk, hard boiled
   4 Tbsp lemon juice
   2 Tbsp balsamic vinegar
   1 tsp Dijon mustard
   1 tsp Worcestershire sauce
   2 Tbsp olive oil
Croutons:
   2 tsp olive oil
   1 clove garlic, halved
   4 1-oz slices Italian bread, cubed
   1 Tbsp chopped fresh parsley
⅓ cup Parmesan cheese

84

1. Crisp lettuce by separating leaves and rinsing well under cold water. Pat dry with paper towels and break into 2-inch pieces. Roll in clean paper towels, place in plastic bag, and seal. Refrigerate until cold and well crisped, about 1 hour.

2. For dressing, combine garlic, pepper, and anchovies in a blender. At high speed, blend until garlic and anchovies are finely chopped. Add egg yolk, lemon juice, vinegar, mustard, and Worcestershire sauce. Blend until mixture is smooth.

3. Turn blender on high and, with machine running, remove center of lid or lid itself. Slowly pour olive oil in a thin, steady stream. Blend until all oil is added and dressing is smooth and creamy. Set aside or refrigerate until ready to add to salad. Do not leave unrefrigerated for more than 1 hour.

4. For croutons, heat olive oil and garlic in medium skillet until oil is hot and garlic is fragrant. Remove pan from heat and cool to room temperature. Discard garlic.

5. Add bread cubes and toss to coat. Sauté over medium-high heat until golden brown. Sprinkle with parsley and cool.

6. To make salad, place crisp lettuce pieces in a medium bowl. Pour dressing over salad and sprinkle with grated Parmesan cheese and croutons. Mix.

LUNCH

1 serving **Pintos and Potatoes**
1 cup **Mastokhiar**
3 finely chopped cashews

63g carb

Pintos and Potatoes

Yield: 6 servings / Serving size: ⅙ recipe

INGREDIENTS
1½ cups dried pinto beans
½ tsp salt
1 potato, peeled and sliced
2 Tbsp lemon juice
2 Tbsp olive oil

METHOD
1. Wash and rinse beans well. Soak beans overnight in enough water to cover.
2. Drain beans and rinse again. Put beans in slow cooker or saucepan and add water to cover by at least 2 inches. Add salt.
3. If using a slow cooker, also add the sliced potato and cook on low for about 12 hours.
4. If cooking on stovetop, simmer until beans are almost tender, about 2 hours, then add sliced potato. Simmer another 45 minutes.
5. Stir in lemon juice and oil before serving.

Mastokhiar

Yield: 2 servings / Serving size: 1 cup

INGREDIENTS
1½ cups low-fat plain yogurt
1 cucumber, peeled and finely chopped
¼ cup raisins
⅛ tsp salt
½ tsp dried or ½ Tbsp chopped fresh mint leaves

METHOD
Mix all ingredients. Chill 1–2 hours before serving.

1 serving **Shrimp and Pea Salad**
2 4-inch bread sticks
1 cup tomato wedges
½ Tbsp Ranch salad dressing
1 slice **Low-Fat Lemon Cheesecake**

Shrimp and Pea Salad

Yield: 4 servings / Serving size: ¼ recipe

INGREDIENTS

1 16-oz pkg. frozen peas, thawed
1 tsp dill
¼ cup chopped red onion
1 cup cooked shrimp, peeled and deveined
2 Tbsp fat-free mayonnaise
½ cup low-fat plain yogurt

METHOD

Mix all ingredients together.

Low-Fat Lemon Cheesecake

Yield: 16 slices / Serving size: 1 slice

INGREDIENTS

¼ cup graham cracker crumbs
16 oz fat-free cream cheese
1 cup sugar
⅔ cup egg substitute
1¾–2 cups plain yogurt cheese (yogurt drained in
  cheesecloth until semisolid)
2 tsp vanilla
1 tsp grated lemon peel
1 Tbsp lemon juice
Sliced oranges, strawberries, and/or kiwis for garnish

METHOD

1. Preheat oven to 350 degrees. Coat a 9-inch springform
   pan with nonstick cooking spray and sprinkle bottom
   with graham cracker crumbs. Refrigerate.
2. In a large bowl, beat cream cheese until smooth.
   Gradually add sugar, beating until smooth. Add
   remaining ingredients except fruit and beat until smooth.
   Pour into pan.
3. Bake 50–60 minutes or until edges are set. (To minimize
   cracking, place a shallow pan half full of hot water on
   lower oven rack while baking.)
4. Remove from oven and cool on a wire rack. Remove
   sides of pan and refrigerate 6 hours or overnight. Top
   with fruit just before serving.

LUNCH

1 cup **Southwestern Veggie Soup**
1 Banana Smoothie:
½ banana
2 oz tofu
1 cup fat-free or low-fat (1%) milk

45

63g carb

Slice peeled banana, place in blender, add tofu and milk, then blend until smooth.

Southwestern Veggie Soup

Yield: 4 servings / Serving size: 1 cup

INGREDIENTS

2 corn tortillas
½ tsp canola oil
⅓ cup chopped onion
⅓ cup chopped green pepper
1 clove garlic, crushed
1½ cups frozen corn
1 medium tomato, chopped
2 cups water
⅓ tsp beef or vegetable bouillon
¼ tsp oregano
1 tsp cornstarch mixed with 1 Tbsp water
1 Tbsp chopped fresh cilantro or parsley leaves
¼ cup mild salsa
1 cup canned pinto beans
1 cup shredded mozzarella cheese
⅛ tsp thyme

METHOD

1. Preheat oven to 400 degrees. Cut tortillas into eighths.
2. Coat nonstick cookie sheet with cooking spray.
3. Bake tortillas for 10 minutes or until crisp.
4. Heat oil and sauté onion, green pepper, and garlic 3–4 minutes.
5. Add remaining ingredients except cheese and thyme and let simmer for 5 minutes.
6. Ladle soup into 4 shallow bowls. Distribute toasted tortilla pieces equally between the bowls.
7. Top each bowl with ¼ cup shredded cheese and a pinch of thyme.

LUNCH

⅓ cup **Hummus with Red Pepper**
1 7-inch whole-wheat pita
1 cup shredded lettuce
1 cup green pepper and tomato salad
1¼ cups cubed watermelon

Hummus with Red Pepper

Yield: 2 cups / Serving size: ⅓ cup

INGREDIENTS

2 cups cooked or canned garbanzo beans, drained (½ cup
   juice reserved)
1 clove garlic
1 Tbsp sesame tahini
2 Tbsp olive oil
1 whole roasted red pepper, seeded (available in jars)
1 Tbsp lemon juice

METHOD

Blend all ingredients in a blender or food processor.

47

67g carb

1 serving **Cucumbers with Dill Dressing**
1 cup Fantastic dry lentil soup,
   reconstituted
2 Tbsp raisins

Cucumbers with Dill Dressing

Yield: 3 servings / Serving size: ¾ cup

INGREDIENTS
Dressing:
   ½ cup wine vinegar
   1 Tbsp canola oil
   1 tsp sugar
   ¼ tsp salt (optional)
   ½ tsp dill
   ¼ tsp pepper
1 cup cucumber slices, ⅛ inch thick
1 cup thinly sliced red onion rings
1 medium tomato, cut into wedges

METHOD
1. Combine dressing ingredients in a large bowl.
2. Add vegetables and mix to coat with dressing.
3. Let stand 15 minutes before serving.

1 serving **Bean Salad**
2 **Whole-Grain Muffins**
1 oz low-fat mozzarella cheese
½ cup pineapple cubes
⅓ cup kiwi slices
½ cup vegetable juice

48

67g carb

Bean Salad

Yield: 6 servings / Serving size: 1 cup

INGREDIENTS

1½ cups fresh green beans
1½ cups fresh yellow beans
1½ cups kidney beans, rinsed and drained
½ cup chopped green pepper
½ cup sliced onions
1 clove garlic, minced
⅔ cup red wine vinegar
1 Tbsp sugar substitute
¼ cup olive oil
½ tsp Worcestershire sauce

METHOD

1. Blanch green and yellow beans. Cool. Mix with kidney beans, peppers, and onions.
2. Mix remaining ingredients and toss with beans. Let stand 1 hour before serving.

Whole-Grain Muffins

Yield: 8 muffins / Serving size: 1 muffin

INGREDIENTS
1 cup whole-wheat flour
1 tsp baking powder
½ tsp salt
1 Tbsp safflower oil
1 egg, beaten
1 cup buttermilk
1 Tbsp molasses

METHOD
1. Preheat oven to 450 degrees.
2. Mix together dry ingredients. Work in oil with a pastry blender.
3. Add egg, buttermilk, and molasses and stir well.
4. Fill lightly greased muffin tins a little more than half full. Bake for 17 minutes. Serve hot.

LUNCH

1 serving **Rigatoni Salad**
¼ cup reduced-fat cottage cheese (4.5%)
9 Triscuits
¾ cup fresh pineapple chunks
½ cup spicy vegetable juice

Rigatoni Salad

Yield: 8 servings / Serving size: ½ cup

INGREDIENTS

1 8-oz box whole-wheat rigatoni
1 cup fat-free Italian dressing
1 cup sliced fresh mushrooms
1 cup chopped green and red peppers
2 Tbsp chopped onions
8 cherry tomatoes for garnish

METHOD

1. Cook rigatoni according to package directions. Drain.
2. Combine all ingredients and garnish with tomatoes. Refrigerate before serving.

Grated Carrot-Raisin Salad
1 Tbsp pine nuts
1 cup Fantastic Five Bean dry soup,
　reconstituted
½ cup vegetable juice

50

72g carb

Grated Carrot-Raisin Salad

Yield: 1 serving

INGREDIENTS
1 medium-sized carrot
2 Tbsp raisins
½ Bartlett pear, peeled and sliced
2 Tbsp fat-free Italian dressing

METHOD
1. Wash and peel carrot. Finely grate carrot in food processor or hand grater.
2. Mix carrots and raisins together. Place mixture in center of plate and surround with pear slices.
3. Drizzle dressing over salad.

LUNCH

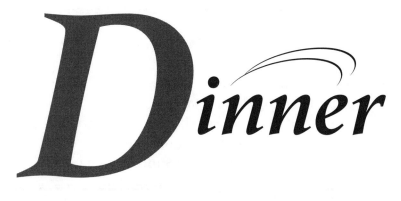

Dinner

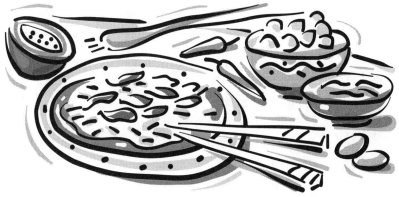

Each dinner in this section has
about 550 calories and includes
2–3 starch servings
1–3 meat or meat substitute
   servings
1–3 vegetable servings
1 fruit serving
1–2 fat servings

Average Fat: 20 grams

Average Carbohydrate: 45 grams

Average Protein: 33 grams

Some menus have 1 fat-free milk
serving instead of 1 meat, 1 starch,
or 1 fruit serving.

No-Fuss Evenings

57g carb

6 oz Stouffer's Macaroni and Cheese (half of a 12-oz pkg.)

1 cup steamed broccoli

Peach melba parfait:

  1 fresh peach, sliced, or ½ cup juice-packed canned peaches

  2 Tbsp Raspberry Sauce (see page 144)

68g carb

4 Mrs. T's frozen pierogies (any type) sautéed in

2 tsp margarine and

2 Tbsp chopped onions

2 oz bratwurst or kielbasa sausage (about a 3-inch piece)

½ cup steamed green beans

½ cup unsweetened applesauce

67g carb

1 Budget Gourmet Beef Stroganoff
1 cup cooked carrots
2 tsp margarine
2 pear halves with
½ cup cottage cheese

64g carb

2 slices Thin-n-Crispy Pizza Hut Pizza
   Supreme (⅓ of 10-inch pizza)
Tossed salad with
1 Tbsp fat-free salad dressing
½ cup fresh mixed fruit

DINNER

5
68g carb

1 serving **Chicken Cacciatore**
⅔ cup cooked brown or white rice
Lettuce with one sliced orange and sliced
   red onion to taste
Dressing:
   2 tsp oil
   2 tsp vinegar

Chicken Cacciatore

Yield: 4 servings / Serving size: ¼ recipe

INGREDIENTS

1 lb cubed boneless skinless chicken breast
1 cup chopped onion
½ cup chopped green pepper
½ cup chopped celery
1 28-oz can chopped stewed tomatoes
½ cup water, divided
1 clove garlic, minced
1 Tbsp minced fresh parsley
Dash oregano
1 Tbsp cornstarch

METHOD

1. Brown pieces of chicken in a nonstick skillet.
2. Add vegetables, ¼ cup water, and spices. Cover and simmer 1 hour.
3. Mix cornstarch with remaining water and add to skillet, stirring until gravy thickens.

DINNER

6

60g carb

1 serving **Shrimp Skewers**
⅔ cup cooked brown or white rice
½ cup sugar-free gelatin cubes with
2 Tbsp whipped topping

Shrimp Skewers

Yield: 1 serving (3 skewers)

INGREDIENTS

6 oz (about 9) large shrimp, peeled and deveined
3 cherry tomatoes
3 pearl onions, peeled
3 1-inch pieces green pepper
6 ½-inch slices zucchini
3 whole mushrooms, cleaned
¾ cup pineapple chunks packed in juice
2 Tbsp fat-free Italian salad dressing

METHOD

1. Alternate shrimp, vegetables, and pineapple on 3 skewers.
2. Broil or grill about 5 minutes on each side or until done. Baste with Italian dressing while cooking. Serve over rice.

DINNER

1 Chicken Taco
⅓ cup refried beans
Fresh vegetable relish tray
1 serving **Pears Filled with Strawberry Cream Cheese**

62g carb

Chicken Tacos

Yield: 12 tacos / Serving size: 1 taco

INGREDIENTS
2 lb boneless skinless chicken breast
½ cup low-sodium, low-fat chicken broth
½ onion, sliced
1 pkg. taco seasoning mix
1½ cups water
12 6-inch flour tortillas
6 oz shredded reduced-fat cheddar cheese
2 cups shredded lettuce
1½ cups chopped tomato
½ cup chopped onion
1 cup salsa (optional)

METHOD
1. Boil chicken in broth and onion for 20 minutes or until done. Remove chicken and cut into small pieces.
2. Return chicken to skillet and add taco seasoning and water.
3. Bring to a boil, then simmer to desired consistency (10–15 minutes).
4. Heat tortillas in microwave or iron skillet. Place ¹⁄₁₂ cooked chicken in the center of each tortilla. Top with ¹⁄₁₂ cheese, lettuce, tomato, and onion. Roll up.

Pears Filled with Strawberry Cream Cheese

Yield: 2 servings / Serving size: ½ pear with 2 oz cream cheese

INGREDIENTS
4 oz low-fat cream cheese
2 fresh strawberries, sliced
¼ tsp brown sugar substitute
1 pear, unpeeled and halved
1 tsp lemon juice

METHOD
1. Combine cream cheese, strawberries, and brown sugar substitute in food processor or blender. Blend until smooth.
2. Spread each pear half with lemon juice, then top with half of the cream cheese mixture.

DINNER

1 serving **Kung Pao Chicken** topped with
6 cashews, chopped
⅔ cup cooked rice
1 cup cooked Chinese kale
1 tsp margarine
1 cup melon balls

59g carb

Kung Pao Chicken

Yield: 4 servings / Serving size: ¼ recipe

INGREDIENTS

1 tsp rice wine vinegar
1 egg white
1 Tbsp cornstarch
2 Tbsp canola oil, divided
12 oz boneless skinless chicken, diced
1 clove garlic, minced
1 green onion, chopped
2 red chili peppers, chopped
1 slice fresh ginger
1½ tsp salt
½ tsp sugar
Chinese hot sauce, if desired
1 Tbsp cooking wine

METHOD

1. In a small bowl, combine rice wine, egg white, cornstarch, and 1 Tbsp oil. Add chicken and toss to coat.
2. Spray wok with nonstick cooking spray. Stir-fry chicken until done.
3. Remove chicken and clean wok. Spray again with nonstick cooking spray. Add remaining 1 Tbsp oil. Heat oil and sauté garlic, onion, chili peppers, ginger, salt, sugar, and hot sauce. Add wine and chicken. Stir. Serve over rice.

2 slices Nutty Rice Loaf
Tossed salad with
2 Tbsp reduced-fat salad dressing
1¼ cups watermelon cubes

59g carb

Nutty Rice Loaf

Yield: 6 servings / Serving size: 1 slice

INGREDIENTS
1½ cups cooked brown rice
1 cup shredded zucchini
¼ cup chopped onion
½ cup wheat germ
¼ cup chopped walnuts
1 cup shredded low-fat cheddar cheese
2 eggs
¼ cup egg substitute
1 tsp thyme
1 tsp marjoram
¼ tsp pepper

METHOD
1. Preheat oven to 350 degrees. Spray a 9- by 5-inch loaf pan with nonstick cooking spray.
2. Combine all ingredients. Pack into loaf pan.
3. Bake for 40–45 minutes or until brown on edges and firm to the touch.
4. Cut into slices. Serve hot or at room temperature.

DINNER

10

65g carb

1 Crab Cake
½ cup green peas
½ cup steamed carrots
1 Tbsp reduced-fat margarine
1 3-inch slice French bread
Tossed salad with
2 Tbsp Parmesan cheese and
2 Tbsp reduced-fat salad dressing
1 baked apple with
Dash cinnamon

Crab Cakes

Yield: 4 servings / Serving size: 1 crab cake

INGREDIENTS

½ lb lump crab meat, flaked
1 Tbsp Dijon mustard
1 Tbsp reduced-fat
   margarine, melted
1 egg, lightly beaten
2 tsp lemon juice

1 tsp Worcestershire sauce
Pinch cayenne pepper
2 dashes Tabasco sauce
½ cup soft bread crumbs
Lemon wedges (optional)

METHOD

1. Preheat oven to 400 degrees. Spray baking sheet with nonstick cooking spray.
2. Combine crab meat, mustard, margarine, egg, lemon juice, Worcestershire sauce, and seasonings. Add 2–4 Tbsp bread crumbs to bind.
3. Shape into 4 cakes (½ cup mixture for each). Roll in remaining bread crumbs; place on cookie sheet.
4. Bake for 20–25 minutes or until lightly browned, turning crab cakes over halfway through cooking time. Serve with lemon wedges, if desired.

DINNER

½ Greek Florentine Pizza
1 cup tossed salad
1 Tbsp fat-free salad dressing
⅔ cup fat-free artificially sweetened lemon
yogurt
1 granola bar

11

77g carb

Greek Florentine Pizza

Yield: 2 servings / Serving size: ½ pizza

INGREDIENTS

1 5-oz Boboli pizza crust
1 tsp olive oil
1 cup frozen spinach, thawed and squeezed dry
2 tsp minced garlic
¼ cup meatless pizza sauce
1 tsp Italian seasoning
1 Tbsp sesame seeds
1 plum tomato, sliced
2 oz feta cheese, crumbled

METHOD

1. Preheat oven to 425 degrees.
2. Heat nonstick skillet. Add oil, spinach, and garlic. Sauté until hot throughout. Remove from heat.
3. Spread sauce on crust. Sprinkle with herbs.
4. Arrange spinach in a circle on crust. Sprinkle with sesame seeds. Arrange sliced tomatoes in a circle. Crumble cheese on top. Bake 15 minutes.

DINNER

12

55g carb

1 serving **Oven-Fried Fish**
½ cup corn
½ cup Italian green beans with pimiento
    garnish and
1 tsp margarine
1 cup cabbage slaw with
Diced green pepper and shredded carrots
1 Tbsp reduced-fat salad dressing
Sugar-free orange gelatin with
    ½ cup sliced juice-packed peaches or
¼ cup orange sherbet

Oven-Fried Fish

Yield: 4 servings / Serving size: 4 oz

INGREDIENTS

1 lb fish fillets (cut into 4 pieces)
2 cups corn flakes
½ tsp each onion powder, oregano, basil, and paprika
1 tsp Parmesan cheese
¼ cup evaporated fat-free milk
4 tsp canola oil

METHOD

1. Preheat oven to 500 degrees.
2. Roll cornflakes into fine crumbs between layers of waxed paper. Add spices.
3. Pour milk into shallow pan. Dip fish in milk, then crumbs.
4. Arrange fish on nonstick baking sheet. Sprinkle oil over fish.
5. Bake for 10 minutes.

2 Stuffed Zucchini halves
⅔ cup cooked brown rice
5 dry-roasted unsalted peanuts

13

65g carb

Stuffed Zucchini

Yield: 4 servings / Serving size: 2 zucchini halves

INGREDIENTS

4 whole zucchini, about
  7 inches long each
1 Tbsp olive oil
1 cup chopped onion
1½ cups chopped green
  pepper
2 cups sliced mushrooms
1 10-oz pkg. frozen spinach,
  thawed
¼ cup chopped pimiento

2 large eggs
½ cup bread crumbs
1 tsp garlic powder
1 tsp onion powder
¼ tsp nutmeg
2 Tbsp thyme
1 15-oz can Italian-style
  tomato sauce
6 oz shredded Swiss cheese

METHOD

1. Preheat oven to 350 degrees.
2. Cut zucchini in half lengthwise and scoop out some of
   the insides to form a shell. Steam shell for 2–3 minutes,
   drain well, and cool.
3. Sauté onion, green pepper, and mushroom in oil until
   soft. Cool.
4. Drain thawed spinach of extra water. Mix spinach, onion,
   pepper, and mushroom with pimiento, eggs, bread
   crumbs, garlic powder, onion powder, nutmeg, and thyme.
5. Fill zucchini shells with stuffing and place in a baking
   dish. Cover with tomato sauce and Swiss cheese.
6. Bake for 15–20 minutes until cheese is melted and sauce
   bubbles.

DINNER

111

14

64g carb

1 serving **Chicken-Fried Steak with Pan Gravy**
1/2 cup mashed potatoes
1 cup green beans
Dinner roll
1 tsp margarine
1 orange

Chicken-Fried Steak with Pan Gravy

Yield: 4 servings / Serving size: 4 oz

INGREDIENTS
1 lb boneless round steak, pounded thin
1 egg, beaten with 1 Tbsp water
1/2 tsp garlic powder
1/4 tsp pepper
1/4 cup flour
1 1/2 Tbsp canola oil
1 Tbsp water
Gravy:
   2 Tbsp flour
   1/2 cup water
   1/2 cup fat-free milk

DINNER

METHOD

1. Trim fat from steak and cut into 4 pieces.
2. Combine garlic powder and pepper. Sprinkle seasonings on both sides of steak.
3. Dredge in flour and shake off excess; dip in egg and again in flour. Heat oil in skillet.
4. Brown both sides of meat in oil, turning only once. Reduce heat to low. Cook for 10–15 minutes or until juices run clear. Add water to skillet, cover, and cook for 5 minutes.
5. Remove steak to heated plate. Add flour to drippings; when light brown, stir in water and milk, whisking until it thickens into a gravy. Add more water if gravy is too thick.
6. Return steaks to skillet; simmer gently until ready to serve.

15

55g carb

4 oz broiled fish (haddock, halibut, or
   salmon)
Lemon wedge
½ cup steamed green beans and onions
1 cup baked acorn squash
1 whole-wheat dinner roll
1 Tbsp reduced-fat margarine
Tossed salad with
2 Tbsp reduced-fat salad dressing
1 **Gelatin Fruit Parfait**

Gelatin Fruit Parfait

Yield: 1 serving

INGREDIENTS

1 pkg. (4-serving size) sugar-free gelatin
½ cup sliced fresh fruit
2 Tbsp whipped topping
Dash nutmeg or cinnamon (optional)

METHOD

1. Prepare gelatin according to package directions. Remove
   ½ cup for this dessert.
2. Alternate layers of fruit and gelatin in parfait glass.
3. Garnish with whipped topping and dash of nutmeg or
   cinnamon, if desired.

DINNER

16

74g carb

1 serving **Crustless Spinach Quiche**
2 3-inch slices French bread
1 cup cooked carrots
2 tsp margarine
Tossed salad with
2 Tbsp reduced-fat salad dressing
1 cup cantaloupe cubes

Crustless Spinach Quiche

Yield: 6 servings / Serving size: ⅙ pie

INGREDIENTS
1 10-oz pkg. frozen chopped spinach, thawed and drained
1 cup shredded part-skim mozzarella cheese
4 eggs plus 2 egg whites, lightly beaten, or 1½ cups egg
   substitute
1 Tbsp grated onion
¼ tsp nutmeg

METHOD
1. Preheat oven to 350 degrees.
2. Mix all ingredients and transfer to an 8-inch pie plate
   coated with nonstick cooking spray.
3. Bake 30 minutes or until knife inserted in center comes
   out clean. Serve hot or cold.

DINNER

17

64g carb

1 baked pork chop or 2 small lamb chops
½ cup cooked noodles
1 whole-wheat dinner roll
2 tsp margarine
1 serving **Crisp Red Cabbage**
½ cup fresh fruit salad

Crisp Red Cabbage

Yield: 6 servings / Serving size: ½ cup

INGREDIENTS
4 cups (about ¾ lb) shredded red cabbage
2 apples, cored and cut into wedges
¼ cup red wine vinegar
2 Tbsp brown sugar
¼ tsp salt
¼ tsp nutmeg

METHOD
1. Place cabbage, apples, vinegar, and brown sugar in saucepan over medium heat. Mix well.
2. Cover and simmer about 10 minutes until cabbage is tender-crisp.
3. Add salt and nutmeg. Mix well. Serve warm.

DINNER

18

64g carb

1 serving **Sally's Hawaiian Chicken**
²⁄₃ cup cooked brown or white rice
1 cup oriental mixed vegetables (frozen variety), stir-fried with
2 tsp olive oil
1 large kiwi fruit

Sally's Hawaiian Chicken

Yield: 8 servings / Serving size: 4 oz

INGREDIENTS
2 lb boneless skinless chicken breast
½ cup low-sodium, low-fat chicken broth
1 20-oz can chunk pineapple packed in juice, undrained
1 cup sliced mushrooms
½ cup chopped bell pepper
1 medium onion, chopped
½ cup water
2 Tbsp lite soy sauce
2 tsp chicken bouillon powder
½ tsp ginger

METHOD
1. Preheat oven to 375 degrees.
2. Brown chicken in nonstick skillet for 3 minutes on each side.
3. Combine all ingredients in large baking dish.
4. Bake uncovered for 30 minutes or until chicken is cooked.

DINNER

1 serving **Vegetarian Lasagna**
Tossed salad with
2 Tbsp reduced-fat salad dressing
1 small nectarine

19

68g carb

Vegetarian Lasagna

Yield: 6 servings / Serving size: 4½- by 4-inch piece

INGREDIENTS

6 lasagna noodles
2 qt water
2 Tbsp canola oil
1 cup chopped onion
1½ cups carrots cut on the diagonal
1 Tbsp minced garlic
2 cups meatless spaghetti sauce (about 1 15-oz jar)
½ cup water
2 tsp basil
1 tsp oregano
2 eggs
2 cups low-fat cottage cheese
4 Tbsp Parmesan cheese
1 10-oz pkg. frozen chopped spinach, thawed and drained
1 cup sliced mushrooms
1 cup quartered and sliced zucchini
¼ cup sliced black olives (optional)
1 cup shredded fat-free mozzarella cheese

DINNER

METHOD

1. Cook lasagna noodles in boiling water about 12 minutes. Drain, rinse, and cover with cold water.
2. Heat oil in saucepan. Add onion, carrots, and garlic. Sauté until carrots are tender, about 10 minutes.
3. Add spaghetti sauce, water, basil, and oregano. Bring to a simmer.
4. Beat eggs and blend in cottage cheese, Parmesan cheese, and vegetables.
5. Preheat oven to 350 degrees.
6. Spread a thin layer of sauce over bottom of 9- by 13-inch baking pan. Cover with a layer of noodles. Spoon half of cheese-vegetable mixture over noodles. Cover with half of sauce. Repeat.
7. Cover with foil and bake for 35 minutes.
8. Remove foil. Arrange olive slices over top and sprinkle with mozzarella cheese. Bake uncovered about 15 minutes, or until center is bubbly.
9. Let stand about 10 minutes to set layers. Cut into 6 pieces.

DINNER

20

64g carb

1 serving **Oven-Fried Chicken**
1 cup mashed potatoes (made with fat-free
   milk) with
2 Tbsp prepared gravy
1 cup steamed green beans
1 **Baked Apple I**

Oven-Fried Chicken

Yield: 2 servings / Serving size: 1 breast half

INGREDIENTS
6 saltine crackers, crushed
2 tsp Parmesan cheese
¼ tsp pepper
⅛ tsp each: basil, celery seed, onion powder, oregano, and
   paprika
1 whole boneless skinless chicken breast, cut in half
1½ Tbsp evaporated fat-free milk

METHOD
1. Preheat oven to 400 degrees.
2. Combine cracker crumbs, cheese, and spices in bowl.
3. Dip chicken in evaporated milk and then coat with
   crumb mixture. Place in shallow nonstick roasting pan.
4. Bake for 30 minutes.

Baked Apple I

Yield: 1 serving

INGREDIENTS

1 apple, cored
¼ tsp cinnamon
½ Tbsp raisins
½ can sugar-free lemon-lime soda

METHOD

1. Preheat oven to 350 degrees.
2. Core apple. Sprinkle with cinnamon and raisins and pour soda over apple.
3. Bake for 20–30 minutes.

DINNER

1 serving **Meat Loaf**
1 small baked potato
2 Tbsp low-fat sour cream
½ cup steamed Brussels sprouts
1 cup coleslaw made with
2 Tbsp reduced-fat salad dressing

54g carb

Meat Loaf

Yield: 6 servings / Serving size: 1½-inch slice

INGREDIENTS
1½ lb ground beef
1 cup fine dry bread crumbs
2 eggs
1 8-oz can tomato sauce
½ cup chopped onion
2 Tbsp chopped green pepper
1½ tsp salt
1 medium bay leaf, crushed
Dash thyme
Dash marjoram

METHOD
1. Preheat oven to 350 degrees.
2. Combine all ingredients; mix well.
3. Pat into 9-inch loaf pan.
4. Bake for 1 hour.

22

64g carb

1 serving **Grilled Pork Loin**
2 small new potatoes, boiled
1 slice French bread
1 tsp margarine
Tossed green salad
2 Tbsp reduced-fat salad dressing
¾ cup fresh pineapple

Grilled Pork Loin

Yield: 4 servings / Serving size: ¼ recipe

INGREDIENTS

1 lb boneless center-cut pork loin, trimmed of excess fat
3 Tbsp minced fresh basil
2 large tomatoes, sliced about ½ inch thick

METHOD

1. Cut pork loin into 4 equal cutlets no more than ½ inch thick.
2. Grill or broil pork. When first side is done, turn pork over and place basil and 1 tomato slice on top.
3. Cover grill and continue cooking until pork is done. (If you cannot cover the grill, cutlets can be placed in a microwave after grilling to cook the tomatoes slightly.)
4. Garnish each plate with remaining tomato slices.

DINNER

23

67g carb

1 serving **Orange Roughy Picante**
1 cup cooked Spanish rice
½ cup green beans topped with
1 tsp margarine and
1 Tbsp pine nuts
1¼ cups watermelon, cubed

Orange Roughy Picante

Yield: 4 servings / Serving size: 4 oz

INGREDIENTS
16 oz orange roughy fillet
½ 16-oz jar mild picante sauce
¼ cup chopped onion
¼ cup chopped green pepper
¼ cup sliced mushroom
¼ cup shredded cheddar cheese

METHOD
1. Preheat oven to 350 degrees.
2. Place fish in oven-safe dish. Cover with picante sauce, and sprinkle with onion, green pepper, and mushroom. Cover with cheese.
3. Bake for 15 minutes or until fish flakes easily with a fork.

DINNER

24

68g carb

1 serving **Sausage and Corn Bread Pie**
½ oz shredded reduced-fat cheddar cheese
Tossed salad with
2 Tbsp reduced-fat salad dressing
½ large pear

Sausage and Corn Bread Pie

Yield: 4 servings / Serving size: ¼ recipe

INGREDIENTS

14 oz turkey sausage
1 cup chopped onion
1 clove garlic, crushed
1 28-oz can chopped
   tomatoes, undrained
¼ cup chopped green
   chilies, undrained
¾ cup frozen corn
1 tsp chili powder

⅔ cup cornmeal
¼ cup whole-wheat or
   white flour
1½ tsp baking powder
¼ tsp salt
1 egg, beaten
⅓ cup fat-free or low-fat
   (1%) milk
1 Tbsp canola oil

METHOD

1. Cook sausage, onion, and garlic in a large skillet over medium heat until meat is browned and crumbled.
2. Add tomatoes, chilies, corn, and chili powder and simmer 20 minutes. Spoon mixture into an 8-inch baking dish coated with nonstick cooking spray. Set aside.
3. Preheat oven to 375 degrees.
4. Combine cornmeal, flour, baking powder, and salt in a medium bowl, mixing well.
5. Combine egg, milk, and oil in a small bowl. Add to dry ingredients, stirring just until moistened.
6. Spread corn bread mixture over sausage mixture. Bake for 30–40 minutes or until golden brown.

DINNER

25

83g carb

1 serving **Spinach Manicotti**
2 Tbsp Parmesan cheese
½ dinner roll
1 tsp margarine
Tossed salad
2 Tbsp reduced-fat salad dressing
1 small pear

Spinach Manicotti

Yield: 5 servings / Serving size: ⅕ recipe

INGREDIENTS

10 manicotti shells
2 6-oz cans tomato paste
3 cups water
½ cup finely chopped onion
2 cloves garlic, crushed
½ tsp basil
½ tsp oregano
¼ tsp salt (optional)

¼ tsp pepper
2 10-oz pkgs. frozen
  chopped spinach
2 cups low-fat cottage
  cheese
⅓ cup Parmesan cheese
¼ tsp ground nutmeg
1 tsp chopped fresh parsley

METHOD

1. Cook manicotti shells according to package directions, omitting salt; drain and set aside.
2. Combine next 8 ingredients; cover and cook sauce over low heat for 1 hour.
3. Preheat oven to 350 degrees. Cook spinach according to package directions, omitting salt. Drain; place on paper towels and squeeze until barely moist.
4. Combine spinach, cottage cheese, Parmesan cheese, and nutmeg. Stuff manicotti shells with spinach mixture and arrange in a 13- by 9- by 2-inch baking dish coated with nonstick cooking spray.
5. Pour tomato sauce over manicotti. Bake for 45 minutes. Garnish with parsley.

DINNER

1 serving **Chicken Fajita**
⅓ cup corn
1 medium orange

Chicken Fajita

Yield: 4 servings
Serving size: ½ cup meat plus one tortilla

INGREDIENTS
1 clove garlic, minced
2½ tsp canola oil
2½ tsp lemon juice
1½ Tbsp soy sauce
Dash pepper
2 tsp Mexican seasoning
2 whole boneless skinless chicken breasts, split
1 medium onion, thinly sliced
1 green pepper, thinly sliced
4 flour tortillas

METHOD
1. Make marinade by combining garlic, 1½ tsp oil, lemon juice, soy sauce, pepper, and Mexican seasoning.
2. Cut chicken into thin strips. Add chicken to marinade, toss to coat evenly, and marinate in refrigerator for at least 2 hours. Stir mixture occasionally to recoat meat.
3. In a nonstick skillet, heat 1 tsp oil on medium-high heat. Add chicken, onion, and pepper. Sauté, stirring occasionally, until chicken is no longer pink and onion is slightly brown. Serve on tortillas.

DINNER

27
52g carb

1 serving **Grilled Tuna Steak**
1 cup steamed new potatoes
Fresh spinach salad
2 Tbsp fat-free Italian salad dressing
1 kiwi, sliced

Grilled Tuna Steak

Yield: 6 servings / Serving size: 4 oz (5 oz before cooking)

INGREDIENTS
½ cup canola oil
¼ cup lemon juice
2 tsp salt
½ tsp Worcestershire sauce
¼ tsp white pepper
⅛ tsp hot pepper sauce
2 lb yellowfin tuna steaks, fresh or frozen, cut into 6 pieces
Paprika

METHOD
1. Combine all ingredients except tuna and paprika. Baste fish with sauce and sprinkle with paprika.
2. Grill tuna about 4 inches from moderately hot coals for 5–6 minutes. Turn, baste with sauce, and sprinkle with paprika; cook 4–5 minutes longer or until tuna has a slightly pink center.

DINNER

28

69g carb

1 serving **Turkey Polynesian**
⅔ cup cooked brown or white rice
Tossed salad
2 Tbsp reduced-fat salad dressing
½ cup sugar-free gelatin with
2 Tbsp whipped topping

Turkey Polynesian

Yield: 4 servings / Serving size: ¼ recipe

INGREDIENTS

2 tsp cornstarch
2 tsp water
1 tsp lite soy sauce
¾ tsp salt (optional)
12 oz uncooked boneless
  skinless turkey breast,
  cubed
½ cup sliced onions
1 Tbsp canola oil, divided

⅔ cup sliced celery
4 oz water chestnuts,
  drained and sliced
⅔ cup snow peas
⅔ cup undrained pineapple
  chunks packed in juice
  (reserve ⅔ cup juice)
⅓ cup mandarin oranges,
  drained

METHOD

1. In small bowl, combine cornstarch, water, soy sauce, and salt. Mix well. Coat turkey cubes with cornstarch mixture.
2. In nonstick skillet over medium heat, sauté onions in half the oil.
3. Add celery, water chestnuts, and snow peas. Cook for 2 minutes. Remove vegetables from skillet.
4. To skillet, add remaining oil and turkey. Sauté until brown. Add sautéed vegetables, pineapple, and juice. Simmer for 10 minutes. Remove from heat. Add oranges. Serve over hot rice.

DINNER

3 oz roasted beef brisket
1 serving **Noodle Pudding**
½ cup sorrel or cooked carrots
1 tsp margarine
1 cup mixed fruit salad

29

61g carb

Noodle Pudding

Yield: 4 servings / Serving size: ½ cup

INGREDIENTS

1 egg
½ Tbsp sugar
Dash nutmeg
⅛ tsp cinnamon
1¼ cups broad noodles, cooked
½ Tbsp canola oil
½ cup apple juice
¼ cup raisins
1 Tbsp chopped pecans

METHOD

1. Preheat oven to 350 degrees.
2. Beat egg and sugar until fluffy. Add remaining ingredients except nuts.
3. Pour into 8-inch baking pan that has been sprayed with nonstick cooking spray. Sprinkle in nuts.
4. Bake for 40 minutes or until browned.

DINNER

1 serving **Grilled Lobster Tails**
1 medium baked potato
3 Tbsp reduced-fat sour cream
1 cup steamed broccoli
1¼ cups fresh or unsweetened frozen
    strawberries

30

68g carb

Grilled Lobster Tails

Yield: 4 servings / Serving size: 3 oz

INGREDIENTS
2 Tbsp butter
¼ cup white wine
¼ tsp lemon pepper or your favorite seasoning
2 6-oz lobster tails (or 12 oz frozen shelled lobster meat)

METHOD
1. Melt butter and combine with wine (much of the alcohol will evaporate, leaving only the flavor) and seasoning.
2. Cut down the back of the lobster tails and gently spread apart. Baste with sauce. Place on a hot grill and continue to baste frequently. Cook for 8 minutes. Baste and turn. Cook for 5 more minutes or until done.

DINNER

1 serving **Chicken with Sun-Dried Tomatoes**
⅔ cup cooked brown or white rice
Tossed salad
2 Tbsp reduced-fat salad dressing
1 medium peach

31

59g carb

Chicken with Sun-Dried Tomatoes

Yield: 4 servings / Serving size: ¼ recipe

INGREDIENTS

4 boneless skinless chicken breast halves (about 1 lb total), trimmed of cartilage and fat
¼ tsp salt (optional)
¼ tsp freshly ground pepper
1 Tbsp canola oil
1 large shallot, minced
⅔ cup low-sodium, low-fat chicken broth
½ cup dry white wine
⅛ tsp marjoram
¼ cup chopped sun-dried tomatoes, rehydrated in small bowl water

DINNER

METHOD

1. Cut each chicken breast half into 6 equal parts. Sprinkle with salt and pepper.
2. Sauté chicken in oil over moderate heat, turning, until the chicken is just opaque throughout, 4–5 minutes.
3. Remove chicken with a slotted spoon. Add shallot to the skillet and sauté, stirring until softened, about 1 minute. Add broth, wine (much of the alcohol will evaporate, leaving only the flavor), marjoram, and tomatoes.
4. Bring to a boil over moderate heat and cook, uncovered, for 5 minutes, stirring occasionally.
5. Return the chicken to the skillet. Simmer, gently spooning the sauce over the chicken, until heated through. Simmer until sauce is reduced by half.

DINNER

1 serving **Corn Soufflé**
½ cup steamed carrots
1 cup steamed green beans
1 tsp margarine
1 Crispbread cracker
½ cup fat-free milk

32

76g carb

Corn Soufflé

Yield: 2 servings / Serving size: ½ recipe

INGREDIENTS
2 tsp reduced-fat margarine
2 Tbsp flour
1 cup fat-free milk
1 tsp garlic powder
1 tsp tarragon
3 eggs, separated
2 cups canned corn, drained

METHOD
1. Preheat oven to 350 degrees.
2. Melt margarine in medium saucepan over low heat. Add flour and stir until smooth. Cook 1 minute, stirring constantly. Gradually add milk and cook over medium heat, stirring constantly, until thick and bubbly. Stir in garlic powder and tarragon.
3. In a large bowl, beat egg yolks until thick. Gradually stir about one-quarter of white sauce into yolks. Add remaining sauce and stir in corn.
4. Beat egg whites until stiff. Gently fold into corn mixture. Spoon mixture into a small 1½-qt soufflé dish that has been coated with cooking spray.
5. Bake for 50 minutes or until puffed and golden. Serve immediately.

DINNER

33

57g carb

1 serving **Herbed Pork Kabobs**
⅔ cup cooked brown and wild rice mixture
½ cup cooked broccoli
1 tsp margarine
1 cup sliced tomato sprinkled with basil and
   rice wine vinegar
½ small mango

Herbed Pork Kabobs

Yield: 4 servings / Serving size: 4-oz skewer

INGREDIENTS

1 lb pork tenderloin, cut
   into 1½ inch cubes
¼ cup dry white wine
¾ tsp dried marjoram,
   divided
¾ tsp dried rosemary, divided

1 garlic clove, minced
3 Tbsp margarine, softened
¼ tsp salt (optional)
Pinch pepper
Lemon wedges

METHOD

1. Combine pork cubes, wine (much of the alcohol will
   evaporate, leaving only the flavor), ¼ tsp marjoram, ¼
   tsp rosemary, and garlic in medium bowl; toss to coat.
   Let stand at room temperature for 20 minutes.
2. Cream together margarine, ½ tsp marjoram, ½ tsp
   rosemary, salt, and pepper.
3. Drain pork; reserve marinade. Beat marinade into
   margarine mix.
4. Set oven to broil. Thread pork on 4 skewers.
5. Place on a wire rack over a shallow baking dish. Broil
   4 inches from heat, turning frequently and basting
   occasionally with herb-butter mix. Brown meat on all
   sides. Serve with lemon wedges.

DINNER

1 serving **Hearty Bean Stew** topped with
1½ oz shredded part-skim mozzarella cheese
Tossed salad
2 Tbsp reduced-fat salad dressing
½ cup light cranberry juice cocktail

Hearty Bean Stew

Yield: 4 servings / Serving size: 1 cup

INGREDIENTS

1 15½-oz can kidney beans, undrained
1 15-oz can garbanzo beans, undrained
1½ cups water
1 medium potato, peeled, quartered lengthwise, and diced
½ cup thinly sliced carrots
¼ cup chopped onion
1 6-oz can tomato paste
1 tsp chili powder
½ tsp salt (optional)
½ tsp crushed dried basil
⅛ tsp garlic powder

METHOD

1. In a Dutch oven, combine all ingredients. Bring to boil; reduce heat.
2. Cover and simmer 30 minutes or until vegetables are tender.

DINNER

1 serving **Pork Dijon**
⅔ cup cooked brown rice
1 cup steamed French-cut green beans with
1 tsp margarine
1¼ cups fresh strawberries with
3 Tbsp reduced-fat sour cream

35

58g carb

Pork Dijon

Yield: 4 servings / Serving size: ¼ recipe

INGREDIENTS
1 lb pork tenderloin
2 tsp olive oil
1 cup chicken broth
2 Tbsp Dijon mustard
1 Tbsp cornstarch

METHOD
1. Cut tenderloin into medallions. Sauté medallions in hot oil in a nonstick frying pan until brown.
2. Mix together chicken broth, mustard, and cornstarch. Pour over medallions.
3. Cook, stirring sauce until thickened; cover and simmer until pork is done. Divide into 4 equal portions.

DINNER

1 serving **Chicken Okra Gumbo**
½ cup cooked broccoli with
1 tsp margarine
2 halves pears packed in juice

36

57g carb

Chicken Okra Gumbo

Yield: 4 servings / Serving size: ¼ recipe

INGREDIENTS

2 whole boneless skinless chicken breasts, cut into chunks
¼ cup flour
Salt to taste (optional)
Pepper to taste
1 Tbsp canola oil
1 lb fresh okra, chopped
1 tomato, chopped
1 medium onion, chopped
4 cups plus 2 Tbsp water
1 tsp Old Bay seasoning
2 tsp cornstarch

METHOD

1. Dredge chicken with mixture of flour, salt, and pepper. In a stockpot, heat oil. Sauté chicken, okra, tomato, and onion until chicken is brown, about 5 minutes.
3. Stir in 4 cups water and Old Bay. Whisk 2 Tbsp water and cornstarch in small bowl, then stir into gumbo. Cook until thickened, 5–10 minutes. Cook for about 30 minutes or until flavors blend.

1 serving **Tamale Pie**
Tossed salad with
Rice or red vinegar and
2 Tbsp shredded Mexican cheese
1 small apple

37

73g carb

Tamale Pie

Yield: 4 servings / Serving size: ¼ recipe

INGREDIENTS

¾ lb lean ground beef
¼ cup chopped green
  pepper
¼ cup chopped onion
½ tsp Mexican seasoning

1 cup canned diced tomatoes,
  drained (reserve 1½ Tbsp
  juice)
¾ cup frozen corn
4 Tbsp green chilies
1 pkg. corn bread mix
Paprika

METHOD

1. Sauté meat, peppers, onions, and seasoning together.
2. Add remaining ingredients except corn bread mix and
   paprika and simmer until well heated and flavors blend,
   about 30 minutes. Stir occasionally.
3. Preheat oven to 375 degrees. Place filling mixture in
   an 8-inch-square baking pan coated with nonstick
   cooking spray.
4. Prepare corn bread batter according to package
   instructions, then divide 1 cup batter into 4 equal
   portions. Spoon each portion about 2 inches apart over
   the warm meat mixture.
5. Bake for 30–40 minutes or until corn bread is done.
   Sprinkle top with paprika, and serve.

DINNER

38

64g carb

1 serving **Bay Scallops Parmesan**
1 small baked potato
2 Tbsp reduced-fat sour cream
½ cup steamed zucchini
1 tsp margarine
1 slice **Chocolate Angel Food Cake**
1¼ cups strawberries, fresh or frozen, unsweetened

Bay Scallops Parmesan

Yield: 4 servings / Serving size: ¼ recipe

INGREDIENTS

2 Tbsp margarine
1 clove garlic, chopped
1 Tbsp white wine
2–4 Tbsp lemon juice (to taste)
1½ lb bay scallops (shrimp or lobster chunks may be substituted)
⅓ cup Parmesan cheese

METHOD

1. Set oven to broil.
2. Place margarine in microwave-safe dish and melt. Add garlic, wine (much of the alcohol will evaporate, leaving only the flavor), lemon, and scallops. Microwave on high for 4 minutes, stirring once after 2 minutes.
3. Place scallops on an individual serving dish that is oven-proof. Sprinkle with Parmesan cheese and place under broiler until cheese is browned.

Chocolate Angel Food Cake

Yield: 32 ½-inch slices / Serving size: 1 slice

INGREDIENTS

1 14½-oz angel food cake mix
¼ cup sifted unsweetened cocoa
¼ tsp chocolate flavoring
1 Tbsp sifted powdered sugar

METHOD

1. Combine flour packet from cake mix with cocoa.
   Prepare cake according to package directions.
2. Fold chocolate flavoring into batter. Bake cake according
   to package directions.
3. Sprinkle cooled cake with powdered sugar.

DINNER

1 serving **Seafood Boil**
Tossed salad with
2 Tbsp reduced-fat French dressing
1 roll
1 tsp margarine
⅓ cup fat-free frozen yogurt

39

53g carb

Seafood Boil

Yield: 8 servings / Serving size: ⅛ recipe

INGREDIENTS

1 Tbsp shrimp boil or other seafood seasoning
8 small-to-medium new potatoes
16 oz turkey kielbasa sausage, cut in ½-inch slices
8 5-inch corn cobettes
1 lb fresh shrimp, shelled and deveined

METHOD

1. In a large pot, bring 1 inch of water and seasonings to a boil.
2. Add potatoes and sausage; cook 15 minutes.
3. Add corn; cook 10 minutes.
4. Add shrimp; cook 10 minutes.

DINNER

1 serving **Mike's Veal**
1 cup cooked pasta (angel hair or
   vermicelli)
Tossed salad with
2 Tbsp reduced-fat Italian dressing
¾ cup mixed melon pieces, orange
   segments, and banana slices

40

80g carb

Mike's Veal

Yield: 4 servings / Serving size: ¼ recipe

INGREDIENTS
1 lb veal for scallopini
¼ cup whole-wheat flour
2 cloves garlic, finely chopped
1 Tbsp olive oil
8 oz sliced mushrooms
½ cup wine (red or white)
4 Roma tomatoes, diced

METHOD
1. Pound veal to tenderize, and divide into 4 pieces.
   Dust lightly with flour. Sauté garlic in oil, then lightly
   brown veal.
2. Remove veal and sauté mushrooms for a few minutes.
3. Add wine, veal, and tomatoes.
4. Cover and heat 2 minutes, then serve.

DINNER

41

57g carb

1 serving **Vegetable Stir-Fry**
5 reduced-fat Triscuits
1 serving **Light and Creamy Yogurt Pie**
with
2 Tbsp Raspberry Sauce

Blend 1 cup raspberries with 2 Tbsp orange juice and 2 packets sugar substitute.

Vegetable Stir-Fry

Yield: 4 servings / Serving size: ¼ recipe

INGREDIENTS

2 Tbsp olive oil
1 small onion, sliced
1 red pepper, thinly sliced
½ Tbsp grated fresh ginger
1 cup broccoli florets
1 lb tofu, drained and cubed
1 cup cooked rotini pasta
4 oz Parmesan cheese

METHOD

1. Heat nonstick skillet or wok to medium high. Add oil and onion and stir-fry 2 minutes.
2. Add pepper and stir-fry 1 minute more.
3. Add ginger, broccoli, and tofu and stir-fry 2 minutes more.
4. Add spaghetti and stir-fry until mixture is thoroughly heated.
5. Top each serving with 2 oz Parmesan cheese.

DINNER

Light and Creamy Yogurt Pie

Yield: 8 slices / Serving size: ⅛ recipe

INGREDIENTS

1 cup low-fat whipped topping
1 cup fat-free artificially sweetened strawberry yogurt
2 cups sliced strawberries or 1½ cups other fruit
1 store-bought 9-inch graham cracker crust

METHOD

1. Fold yogurt into whipped topping and add most of the fruit.
2. Fill crust. Garnish with remaining fruit.
3. Chill or freeze. May be served frozen.

DINNER

42

54g carb

1 serving **New England Chicken Croquettes**
⅓ cup cooked brown rice
½ cup cooked spinach
1 tsp margarine
1 cup fresh raspberries

New England Chicken Croquettes

Yield: 8 croquettes / Serving size: 2 croquettes

INGREDIENTS

2 Tbsp margarine
2 Tbsp flour
1 cup fat-free milk
1 tsp Worcestershire sauce
½ tsp chervil
½ tsp salt
⅛ tsp white pepper
2 cups finely chopped cooked chicken
⅔ cup bread crumbs
2 eggs, lightly beaten

METHOD

1. Preheat oven to 375 degrees.
2. Melt margarine over low heat; stir in flour until smooth. Add milk gradually, whisking until smooth; add Worcestershire sauce, chervil, salt, pepper, and chicken. Cool.
3. When cold, form into 8 balls, using ⅓ cup mixture per ball.
4. Roll in bread crumbs, egg, and again in bread crumbs.
5. Place on cookie sheet well coated with nonstick cooking spray. Bake for 25–30 minutes or until light golden brown.

1 serving **French Onion Soup**
1 oz French bread
3 oz lean roast beef
1 cup tossed salad
1 Tbsp fat-free salad dressing
1 cup cantaloupe

43

56g carb

French Onion Soup

Yield: 6 servings / Serving size: 1 cup

INGREDIENTS
5 cups thinly sliced onion
2 Tbsp butter or margarine
3 10½-oz cans condensed beef broth
1 qt water
½ tsp salt (optional)
Fresh ground pepper to taste
6 slices French bread, toasted
½ cup shredded Swiss cheese
2 Tbsp Parmesan cheese

METHOD
1. Preheat oven to 400 degrees.
2. Sauté onions slowly in butter until they turn a delicate gold.
3. Add beef broth and water. Cover and simmer gently for 45 minutes. Add salt and pepper.
4. Place in large oven-proof soup tureen or individual bowls. Top with toasted French bread and sprinkle with grated Swiss and Parmesan cheese.
5. Bake for 8 minutes.

DINNER

44

57g carb

1 cup **Hoppin' John**
1 cup **Seasoned Greens**
1 piece corn bread (2 by 2 by 1½ inches)
2 tangerines

Hoppin' John

Yield: 8 servings / Serving size: 1 cup

INGREDIENTS

1 cup raw cow peas (dried field peas) or dried black-eyed
  peas
4 cups water
1 cup uncooked brown rice
4 slices bacon, fried crisp and fat drained
1 medium onion, chopped

METHOD

1. Boil peas in lightly salted water until tender. Drain peas,
   reserving 2 cups liquid.
2. Stir together peas, pea liquid, rice, bacon, and onion.
3. Cook covered for 1 hour or until rice is done.

DINNER

Seasoned Greens

Yield: 8 servings / Serving size: ½ cup

INGREDIENTS

1 large bunch collard, mustard, or turnip greens or 1 lb
   frozen greens
2 fresh center-cut pork chops, trimmed of fat and chopped
Salt, pepper, and hot sauce to taste

METHOD

1. Rinse greens well in water. Cut or tear into small pieces.
2. Place greens and pork in a 2-qt saucepan and cover with
   water. Bring to a boil and cook about 5 minutes.

DINNER

1 slice **Salmon Loaf**
1 cup steamed broccoli
1 small baked potato
2 Tbsp sour cream
1 tsp margarine
1¼ cups strawberries

58g carb

Salmon Loaf

Yield: 4 servings / Serving size: 1 slice

INGREDIENTS

1 15½-oz can salmon, undrained
2 eggs, beaten
2 cups soft bread cubes or ⅓ cup bread crumbs
2 Tbsp fresh chopped parsley
⅛ tsp pepper
1 small onion, chopped
2 Tbsp lemon juice

METHOD

1. Preheat oven to 350 degrees. Generously spray an 8½-by 2½-inch loaf pan with nonstick cooking spray.
2. In a large bowl, flake salmon, removing bones and skin.
3. Add all remaining ingredients and mix well.
4. Press into loaf pan. Bake for 50–60 minutes or until golden brown and toothpick comes out clean.
5. Let stand 5 minutes. Loosen edges and lift out of pan onto serving platter. Cut into 4 slices.

DINNER

1 serving **Picante Tofu and Rice**
6 chopped cashews
Iced Café Mocha (see page 192)
⅓ cup fat-free artificially sweetened fruit-flavored yogurt

46

77g carb

Picante Tofu and Rice

Yield: 1 serving

INGREDIENTS

½ cup chopped red onion
½ cup each chopped green and red peppers
2 Tbsp chopped green chilis
2 tsp minced garlic
6 oz firm tofu, drained and cubed
1 tsp olive oil
⅓ cup uncooked rice
¾ cup pinto beans, rinsed and drained
⅔ cup vegetable broth
⅓ cup picante sauce
1 tsp cumin
¼ tsp chili powder or to taste
½ cup tomato wedges
⅛ avocado, sliced
¼ cup shredded low-fat Monterey Jack cheese

METHOD

1. Sauté onion, peppers, chilis, garlic, and tofu in oil until just tender-crisp.
2. Add rice, beans, broth, and picante sauce. Bring to a boil. Reduce heat, cover, and simmer 15 minutes until rice is tender.
3. Add seasonings. Toss and let stand until liquid is absorbed. Garnish with tomato, avocado, and cheese.

DINNER

1 cup **Broccoli-Corn Chowder**
2 oz shredded reduced-fat cheddar cheese, sprinkled on soup
1 piece sourdough bread
1 tsp margarine
Tossed salad
2–3 Tbsp fat-free salad dressing
½ cup fat-free artificially sweetened frozen yogurt (70 calories/serving)

47

62g carb

Broccoli-Corn Chowder

Yield: 16 servings / Serving size: 1 cup

INGREDIENTS

1 qt fat-free reduced sodium chicken broth
1 10-oz pkg. frozen chopped broccoli
1 lb frozen whole-kernel corn
1½ cups sliced mushrooms

1½ cups chopped onion
¼ cup margarine
¾ cup flour
½ tsp white pepper
2½ cups fat-free milk
¼ cup chopped pimientos

METHOD

1. In a large kettle, combine chicken broth, broccoli, and corn.
2. Bring to a boil. Reduce heat to low and simmer 15 minutes. Set aside.
3. Sauté mushrooms and onion in margarine.
4. Blend flour and pepper into mushroom mixture. Add to broccoli mixture.
5. Add milk and simmer on low heat for about 30 minutes, stirring occasionally.
6. Stir in pimientos before serving.

DINNER

1 serving **Saucy Seafood Stir-Fry**
2 Tbsp Parmesan cheese
⅔ cup cooked brown rice
½ cup Waldorf Salad

48

55g carb

Saucy Seafood Stir-Fry

Yield: 4 servings / Serving size: ¼ recipe

INGREDIENTS

1 tsp canola oil
1 cup broccoli florets
1 cup cauliflower florets
½ cup julienned carrots
¼ cup sliced red peppers
¼ cup sliced green peppers
¼ cup sliced yellow peppers

½ lb shrimp, peeled and
   deveined
½ lb scallops
2 tsp reduced-fat margarine
1 Tbsp reduced-fat
   mayonnaise
Juice of 1 lemon

METHOD

1. Spray a large frying pan or wok with nonstick cooking spray; heat oil to medium-high.
2. Stir-fry broccoli, cauliflower, and carrots about 4 minutes. Then add peppers.
3. Add shrimp to mixture and continue stir-frying until shrimp turn pink. Add scallops and continue stir-frying until scallops turn white. Set aside.
4. Melt margarine in microwave or oven. Whip mayonnaise and melted margarine together until smooth. Add lemon juice.
5. Combine with stir-fry mixture. Toss to coat.

DINNER

49

66g carb

1 cup cooked linguine
1 cup **Clam Sauce**
2 Tbsp Parmesan cheese
Fresh spinach salad:
    Spinach greens
    Red onion rings
    ¼ cup water-packed mandarin orange
        sections, drained
2 Tbsp reduced-fat Catalina dressing

Clam Sauce

Yield: 5 cups / Serving size: 1 cup

INGREDIENTS

2 tsp olive oil
1 cup chopped onion
2 cloves garlic, minced
½ green pepper, chopped
1½ cups sliced mushrooms
3 10-oz cans whole baby
    clams with liquid

1½ cups tomatoes, peeled,
    seeded, and diced
¼ cup low-fat whipping
    cream
Pepper to taste
¾ cup Parmesan cheese

METHOD

1. Heat skillet and add olive oil. Sauté onion, garlic, pepper, and mushrooms.
2. Add clams and liquid. Simmer to reduce liquid by one-third to one-half.
3. Add tomato and cream and simmer until large glossy bubbles form.
4. Season and toss with Parmesan cheese. Serve 1 cup sauce over 1 cup cooked linguine.

DINNER

1 serving **Chicken Curry**
½ cup cooked rice with
1 tsp margarine and parsley
Tossed salad with
2 Tbsp reduced-fat salad dressing
⅓ cup canned unsweetened pineapple cubes

50

63g carb

Chicken Curry

Yield: 6 servings / Serving size: ⅙ recipe

INGREDIENTS

2-inch piece fresh ginger,
  peeled
12 cloves garlic
1 cup plus 2 Tbsp water
2 medium onions, sliced
1 Tbsp canola oil
2-inch piece cinnamon stick
6 whole cloves
3 big cardamom seeds
  (optional)

2 tsp chili powder
1 tsp cumin seed
½ tsp salt (optional)
½ tsp turmeric powder
1 3-lb chicken, skinned and
  cut into serving-size pieces
½ cup fat-free plain yogurt
2 tomatoes, peeled and
  chopped
⅓ cup chopped cilantro

METHOD

1. Make a paste of the ginger, garlic, and 2 Tbsp water.
2. Sauté onion in oil until brown. Add all spices and chicken and yogurt; continue to cook, sprinkling with additional water as required to keep from sticking.
3. Cook until chicken browns (about 10 minutes). Add 1 cup of water and let simmer on low heat for about 45 minutes or until chicken is tender.
4. Add chopped tomato after about 30 minutes. Before serving, add cilantro.

DINNER

1 serving **Prune-Stuffed Tenderloin**
½ baked acorn squash
1 tsp margarine
5 spears steamed asparagus
Tossed salad
2 Tbsp reduced-fat salad dressing

51

63g carb

Prune-Stuffed Tenderloin

Yield: 4 servings / Serving size: ¼ recipe (2½-inch slice)

INGREDIENTS

15 dried pitted prunes, coarsely chopped
⅓ cup chicken broth
¼ cup chopped celery
¼ cup chopped onion
1 tsp canola oil
3 slices multigrain bread, cubed
⅛ tsp poultry seasoning
1 lb pork tenderloin
1 clove garlic, crushed
⅛ tsp fennel seeds
¼ tsp pepper
1 Tbsp margarine, melted

DINNER

METHOD

1. Bring prunes and broth to a boil in a saucepan. Remove from heat and let stand for 10 minutes.
2. Sauté celery and onion in oil until tender.
3. Place bread cubes and poultry seasoning in a large bowl. Toss to mix. Add celery, onions, prunes, and broth. Toss lightly to blend. Add more broth if dressing is too dry.
4. Preheat oven to 500 degrees. Trim excess fat from tenderloin. Cut lengthwise to within ½ inch of each end and almost to the bottom, leaving bottom connected. Open meat and pound sides of pocket to about ¼ inch thickness.
5. Combine garlic, fennel seeds, and pepper, and rub on the inside of the pocket.
6. Spoon stuffing into opening of tenderloin. Press gently to close. Tie tenderloin securely with heavy string at 1-inch intervals.
7. Place tenderloin on a roasting rack coated with vegetable spray. Place rack in roasting pan. Insert meat thermometer into thickest part of tenderloin.
8. Place tenderloin in oven and immediately reduce temperature to 350 degrees. Cook 20 minutes, then brush on margarine and cook an additional 10–15 minutes until meat thermometer reaches 170 degrees.
9. Remove from oven, cover with aluminum foil, and let stand 10 minutes before slicing into 4 equal portions.

DINNER

1 piece **Zucchini Lasagna**
1 cup steamed broccoli
2 tsp margarine
68g carb 1 cup fat-free or low-fat (1%) milk
½ poached pear
2 Tbsp Raspberry Sauce (see page 144)

Zucchini Lasagna

Yield: 9 servings / Serving size: 3- by 3-inch piece

INGREDIENTS

1 16-oz jar marinara sauce
1 8-oz can tomatoes
½ lb (9–12) lasagna noodles
15 oz ricotta cheese
2 large eggs, beaten
½ tsp basil
½ tsp oregano
¼ cup Parmesan cheese
3 cups coarsely grated zucchini
⅛ tsp pepper
2 tsp flour
8 oz shredded mozzarella cheese

METHOD

1. Preheat oven to 350 degrees. Coat a 9-inch-square baking dish with nonstick cooking spray.
2. Combine marinara and tomatoes. Spread ½ cup of the mixture over bottom of dish. Arrange uncooked noodles in dish, breaking off ends to make them fit. Place ends in open spaces.
3. Combine ricotta, eggs, basil, oregano, and Parmesan. Spread over lasagna noodles. Top with more noodles and ½ cup more sauce.
4. Combine zucchini, pepper, and flour. Spoon into baking dish and spread to make a level layer. Top with more lasagna noodles and remaining sauce.
5. Cover dish with foil and place on a rimmed baking sheet. Bake 55–60 minutes or until noodles are tender. Remove foil and sprinkle with mozzarella. Bake 15–20 minutes more until cheese is golden brown (or place under broiler). After removing lasagna from oven, let stand 15 minutes before cutting.

DINNER

1 serving **Brunswick Stew**
1 cup salad greens with
½ cup citrus sections and
56g carb ¼ cup cottage cheese
6 Wheat Thin crackers
Dressing:
  1 Tbsp orange juice
  1 Tbsp vinegar
  2 tsp vegetable oil

Brunswick Stew

Yield: 4 servings / Serving size: 1½ cups

INGREDIENTS

1 cup water
4 medium chicken thighs, skin and fat removed
2 celery stalks, chopped
½ cup chopped onion
1 28-oz can tomatoes and juice
1 cup frozen lima beans
1 cup frozen corn
1 cup cubed potatoes
Salt and pepper to taste

METHOD

1. Combine water, chicken, celery, and onion in a medium saucepan and bring to a boil. Cover and simmer 1½–2 hours to make broth.
2. Remove chicken and chop, discarding bones. Return chicken to broth.
3. Add remaining ingredients and bring to a boil.
4. Cover, reduce heat, and simmer 30–40 minutes or until vegetables are tender.

54

65g carb

1 serving **Chicken Ratatouille**
⅔ cup cooked barley
¾ cup mixed fresh fruit salad, topped with
2 Tbsp fat-free fruit-flavored yogurt

Chicken Ratatouille

Yield: 4 servings
Serving size: 1 breast half and 1½ cups vegetables

INGREDIENTS

4 boneless skinless chicken
  breast halves
1 Tbsp olive oil
1 small eggplant, cubed
2 small zucchini, sliced
1 onion, sliced
½ lb mushrooms, sliced
1 green pepper, sliced

1 large tomato, cubed
½ tsp garlic powder
1 tsp dried parsley
1 tsp basil
1 tsp pepper
½ cup shredded part-skim
  mozzarella cheese

METHOD

1. Sauté chicken in oil about 2 minutes per side.
2. Add eggplant, zucchini, onion, mushrooms, and green pepper. Cook 10 minutes.
3. Add tomato and remaining ingredients except cheese and simmer 3–5 minutes more.
4. Arrange chicken on top of vegetables and sprinkle cheese over chicken. Cook 1 more minute until cheese melts.
5. Serve over barley.

DINNER

1 serving **Yogurt Chicken Paprika**
½ cup cooked egg noodles
½ cup steamed spinach
1 Tbsp reduced-fat margarine
1 serving **Old-Fashioned Banana Pudding**

55

62g carb

Yogurt Chicken Paprika

Yield: 4 servings / Serving size: 1 breast half plus ½ cup sauce

INGREDIENTS

1½ cups chopped onions
1 Tbsp butter
1 Tbsp paprika
4 boneless skinless chicken breast halves
1 cube chicken bouillon
1 cup hot water
1 Tbsp cornstarch
1 cup fat-free plain yogurt

METHOD

1. Sauté onion in butter in large skillet. Blend in paprika. Add chicken and brown well.
2. Dissolve bouillon in 1 cup hot water and add to skillet. Cover and simmer 30–40 minutes until chicken is tender.
3. Dissolve cornstarch in 1 Tbsp cold water. Blend into yogurt. Stir yogurt mixture into skillet, heat slightly, and serve.

DINNER

Old-Fashioned Banana Pudding

Yield: 6 servings / Serving size: ⅓ cup

INGREDIENTS

1 1-oz pkg. sugar-free vanilla pudding
2 cups fat-free or low-fat (1%) milk
12 vanilla wafers
2 large bananas

METHOD

1. Combine pudding mix and milk. Cook over medium heat, stirring frequently, until mixture boils, then remove from heat.
2. Place 2 cookies on bottom of each of 6 custard dishes. Alternate layers of bananas and pudding, starting and finishing with bananas.
3. Chill before serving.

DINNER

2 Stuffed Vegetarian Peppers
2 oz Monterey Jack cheese
½ cup **Italian Fruit Salad**

65g carb

Stuffed Vegetarian Peppers

Yield: 6 servings / Serving size: 2 peppers

INGREDIENTS

2 cups uncooked couscous
4 cups boiling water
6 red peppers
6 yellow peppers
¼ cup minced shallots
¼ cup plus 1 Tbsp olive oil

1 lb asparagus
3 Tbsp tarragon
2 cups peas
½ tsp pepper
½ tsp paprika

METHOD

1. Place couscous in a large bowl and cover with boiling water. Cover with plastic wrap and let sit for 20 minutes.
2. Slice tops off peppers and remove the white membranes and seeds. Steam peppers and their tops for 5–7 minutes until tender.
3. Preheat oven to 350 degrees. Sauté shallots in 1 Tbsp oil until translucent. Chop the tender parts of the asparagus into 1-inch pieces.
4. With a wooden spoon, fluff the couscous and add remaining ingredients, including ¼ cup oil. Mix thoroughly.
5. Stuff the mixture into the peppers, using about ⅔ cup per pepper. Cover with the tops of the peppers. Put the peppers into a large casserole dish with ¼ inch of water at the bottom. Cover and bake for 45 minutes.
6. To serve, discard each pepper top and sprinkle with paprika.

DINNER

Italian Fruit Salad

Yield: 6 servings / Serving size: ½ cup

INGREDIENTS

¼ cup freshly squeezed orange juice
Juice and rind of ¼ lemon
1 apple, unpeeled and cubed
1 pear, unpeeled and cubed
¼ lb seedless grapes
1 peach, peeled and sliced
1 banana, sliced
2 packets sugar substitute (optional)
1 Tbsp orange liqueur (optional)

METHOD

1. Combine orange juice and lemon rind and juice in a large bowl. As you cut fruit, mix it with juice to keep it from discoloring.
2. Add sweetener and orange liqueur to taste. Toss lightly.
3. Cover bowl with plastic wrap and chill at least 2 hours before serving.

DINNER

1 serving **Asian Chicken**
⅓ cup cooked rice or chow mein noodles
Tossed salad with
1 tsp oil and
Vinegar to taste
¾ cup **Fruit Crisp**
1 cup fat-free or low-fat (1%) milk

57

72g carb

Asian Chicken

Yield: 4 servings / Serving size: ¼ recipe

INGREDIENTS

1 Tbsp canola oil
4 chicken thighs, skin and
  fat removed
½ cup dry white wine
¼ cup chopped green onions
¼ cup chopped onion
½ cup sliced celery
1 tsp minced fresh ginger

4 oz (½ 8-oz can) water
  chestnuts, drained and
  rinsed
8 oz mushrooms, sliced
¼ tsp garlic powder
¼ tsp dried red pepper flakes
1 tsp brown sugar
2 Tbsp lite soy sauce
8 oz snow peas, fresh or
  frozen

METHOD

1. Heat oil in large skillet and sauté chicken 3–5 minutes. Remove chicken.
2. Add wine to skillet and scrape pan to deglaze. Add onions, celery, and ginger and sauté until wine is reduced by half, about 5 minutes.
3. Add water chestnuts and mushrooms and sauté 2 minutes.
4. Add seasonings and chicken, cover, and simmer 10 minutes.
5. Add snow peas and cook 5 more minutes.

Fruit Crisp

Yield: 6 servings / Serving size: ¾ cup

INGREDIENTS

3 cups sliced apples
1 16-oz can juice-packed peaches, undrained
½ cup oatmeal
½ cup whole-wheat flour
¾ tsp cinnamon
¾ tsp nutmeg
¾ tsp cornstarch
2 Tbsp reduced-fat margarine

METHOD

1. Preheat oven to 375 degrees.
2. Lightly coat a 9- by 9-inch baking pan with nonstick cooking spray.
3. Put apples and peaches in pan.
4. In a separate bowl, combine remaining ingredients. Stir half of mixture into fruit.
5. Sprinkle remainder of the dry mixture over top of the fruit and bake for 30 minutes.

DINNER

3 Porcupine Meatballs
½ cup steamed carrots
1 cup celery sticks and radishes
8 large Spanish olives
1 Baked Apple II

58

58g carb

Porcupine Meatballs

Yield: 2 servings / Serving size: 3 meatballs

INGREDIENTS
8 oz ground beef
⅔ cup cooked rice
1½ Tbsp dried minced onion
¼ tsp pepper
⅛ tsp oregano
1 cup tomato sauce
1 cup water

METHOD
1. Mix meat, rice, onion, and seasonings until well blended. Form into 6 meatballs.
2. Brown meatballs in skillet on all sides.
3. Drain fat, then add tomato sauce and water. Cover and simmer 15–20 minutes.

DINNER

Baked Apple II

Yield: 2 servings / Serving size: 1 apple

INGREDIENTS

2 small cooking apples
2 tsp margarine
2 tsp 100% fruit currant or grape jelly

METHOD

1. Preheat oven to 350 degrees.
2. Core apples, leaving bottom intact. Place in oven-proof baking dish with ½ inch water.
3. Put 1 tsp margarine and 1 tsp jelly in each apple.
4. Bake for 30 minutes or until tender.
5. Baste with jelly-margarine mixture before serving.

1 serving **Barbecued Chicken**
1 6-inch ear corn on the cob
½ cup steamed broccoli
½ cup carrot sticks
1 slice **Sally Lunn Peach Cake**

59

60g carb

Barbecued Chicken

Yield: 2 servings / Serving size: ½ recipe

INGREDIENTS
2 chicken thighs and 2 chicken legs
½ cup **Barbecue Sauce**

METHOD
1. Marinate raw chicken pieces in barbecue sauce at least 2 hours in the refrigerator, turning occasionally.
2. Cook on outdoor grill until chicken is no longer pink.

Barbecue Sauce

Yield: 4½ cups / Serving size: ¼ cup

INGREDIENTS
1 small onion, minced
2 8-oz cans tomato sauce
2 cups water
¼ cup wine vinegar
¼ cup Worcestershire sauce
1 tsp salt (optional)

2 tsp paprika
2 tsp chili powder
1 tsp pepper
½ tsp cinnamon
⅛ tsp ground cloves

METHOD
1. Combine all ingredients in a saucepan. Bring to a full boil.
2. Reduce heat and simmer for 20 minutes.

DINNER

Sally Lunn Peach Cake

Yield: 1 loaf of 12 slices / Serving size: 1 slice

INGREDIENTS

2 cups sifted flour
3 tsp baking powder
½ tsp salt
1 egg, beaten
¾ cup fat-free or low-fat (1%) milk
½ cup canola oil
¼ cup sugar
4 cups fresh or juice-packed peaches, drained

METHOD

1. Preheat oven to 375 degrees.
2. Sift flour with baking powder and salt.
3. Combine egg, milk, and oil in a large bowl. Add sugar. Stir in dry ingredients. Do not overmix.
4. Pour batter into a loaf pan that has been coated with cooking spray.
5. Bake for 30 minutes.
6. Top each slice with ⅓ cup sliced peaches.

DINNER

3 oz **Fish Creole**
⅔ cup cooked brown or white rice
½ cup green beans
2 tsp margarine
1 peach

60

56g carb

Fish Creole

Yield: 4 servings / Serving size: 3-oz fillet plus sauce

INGREDIENTS
4 3-oz fish fillets
2 Tbsp lemon juice
2 Tbsp finely chopped onion
4 Tbsp reduced-fat margarine, divided
½ cup chopped green peppers
1 cup chopped canned tomatoes, undrained
Pepper to taste
2 tsp flour

METHOD
1. Preheat oven to 350 degrees.
2. Place fish fillets in baking pan coated with nonstick cooking spray.
3. Mix together lemon juice, onion, and 2 Tbsp melted margarine.
4. Pour mixture over fish. Bake uncovered or until fish flakes easily with fork, about 15 minutes.
5. While fish is baking, prepare creole sauce: sauté green pepper in remaining margarine. Add tomatoes and pepper. Stir in flour. Simmer until mixture is heated.

DINNER

1 serving **Bok Choy Sauté** topped with
9 cashews, chopped
⅔ cup cooked brown rice
⅓ cup fresh pineapple chunks mixed with
½ cup fresh strawberries

61

59g carb

Bok Choy Sauté

Yield: 2 servings / Serving size: ½ recipe

INGREDIENTS
1 Tbsp sesame oil
1 clove garlic, crushed
8 oz pork tenderloin, thinly sliced
1 cup sliced shiitake or other mushrooms
1½ cups sliced bok choy, with leaves
4 oz (½ 8-oz can) water chestnuts, drained
1 Tbsp lite soy sauce

METHOD
1. Heat oil in large skillet or wok over medium-high heat and stir-fry garlic 1 minute.
2. Add pork, stirring constantly, and stir-fry 3–5 minutes. Add mushrooms and stir-fry for 1 minute. Add bok choy and water chestnuts and stir-fry 2–3 minutes.
3. Add soy sauce and toss to coat.

DINNER

2 Black Bean Cakes
½ cup **Cilantro Salsa**
1 oz shredded Monterey Jack cheese
½ cup fruit gelatin

62

58g carb

Black Bean Cakes

Yield: 2 servings / Serving size: 2 cakes

INGREDIENTS
1¼ cups cooked black beans
½ cup chopped onion
½ cup chopped fresh cilantro or parsley
2 Tbsp Korean chili-garlic paste or plain tomato paste
1 egg, lightly beaten
2 Tbsp fat-free or low-fat (1%) milk
Salt and pepper to taste
¼ cup dry bread crumbs
2 Tbsp olive oil

METHOD
1. Thoroughly mix all ingredients except bread crumbs
   and olive oil. Add bread crumbs to mixture and form
   into 4 patties.
2. Heat oil in skillet and gently slide patties into skillet.
   Sauté until brown and crisp on both sides.

DINNER

Cilantro Salsa

Yield: 4 servings / Serving size: ½ cup

INGREDIENTS

2 tomatoes, diced
1 small cucumber, peeled and chopped
1 small red onion, diced
½ cup chopped fresh cilantro leaves
1 tsp grated lime peel
1 small green pepper, diced
1–2 dashes hot sauce
Salt and pepper to taste

METHOD

Blend all ingredients to desired chunkiness and chill
overnight.

DINNER

1 serving **Jambalaya**
Tossed salad with
2 Tbsp reduced-fat salad dressing and
2 Tbsp reduced-fat cheddar cheese and
4 pecan halves, chopped
1 cup melon cubes

63

66g carb

Jambalaya

Yield: 4 servings / Serving size: 1½ cups

INGREDIENTS

4 oz lean ham, chopped
1 cup chopped onion
2 celery stalks, chopped
1 medium green pepper, chopped
1 28-oz can tomatoes, undrained
¼ cup tomato paste
1 clove garlic, minced
1 Tbsp minced fresh parsley
¼ tsp thyme
2 whole cloves
1 Tbsp canola oil
⅔ cup uncooked brown or white rice
16 medium-large shrimp, peeled and deveined

METHOD

1. Thoroughly mix all ingredients except shrimp in a slow cooker. Cover and cook on low setting for 7–10 hours.
2. One hour before serving, turn slow cooker to high setting. Stir in uncooked shrimp. Cover and cook until shrimp are pink and tender.

DINNER

2 Hawaiian Kabobs
⅔ cup cooked white rice
Tossed salad
2 Tbsp reduced-fat salad dressing
10 peanuts

64

62g carb

Hawaiian Kabobs

Yield: 4 servings / Serving size: 2 skewers

INGREDIENTS
1 Tbsp lite soy sauce
¼ cup pineapple juice
½ tsp garlic powder
1 tsp ground ginger
½ tsp dry mustard
¼ tsp pepper
2 Tbsp canola oil
14 oz boneless skinless chicken breast, cut into 1-inch cubes
2 cups fresh or juice-packed pineapple chunks, drained
2 medium green peppers, cut into chunks
16 medium mushrooms
8 cherry tomatoes

METHOD
1. Combine first 7 ingredients in a small saucepan and bring to a boil. Reduce heat and simmer 5 minutes. Let cool.
2. Pour mixture into a shallow dish and add chicken, tossing gently to coat. Cover and marinate at least 1 hour in the refrigerator, stirring mixture occasionally.
3. Remove chicken from marinade, reserving marinade. Alternate chicken, pineapple, green pepper, mushrooms, and tomatoes on 8 skewers.
4. Grill over hot coals 20 minutes or until done, turning and basting frequently with marinade.

DINNER

177

65

59g carb

1 serving **Apricot-Glazed Ham**
½ cup **Lightly Scalloped Potatoes**
1 cup steamed green beans
1 slice reduced-calorie whole-wheat bread
1½ Tbsp reduced-fat margarine
½ cup sugar-free lemon gelatin
1 Tbsp whipped topping

Apricot-Glazed Ham

Yield: 4 servings / Serving size: 3 oz ham and ¼ cup glaze

INGREDIENTS
½ cup orange juice
2 Tbsp currants or raisins
1 cup juice-packed apricots, drained
¼ tsp ginger (optional)
12-oz lean ham steak, fat trimmed

METHOD
1. Preheat oven to 350 degrees.
2. Combine orange juice, currants, apricots, and ginger in a small saucepan. Cook over medium heat until thickened, about 8–10 minutes.
3. Place ham slice on baking pan. Pour sauce over ham and bake for about 20 minutes. Divide ham into 4 equal servings.

DINNER

Lightly Scalloped Potatoes

Yield: 8 servings / Serving size: ½ cup

INGREDIENTS
1 clove garlic, minced
¼ cup diced onion
2½ tsp flour
6 oz evaporated fat-free milk
¾ cup fat-free milk
½ tsp salt
¼ tsp red pepper
4½ cups (2½ lb) thinly sliced red potatoes
½ cup shredded reduced-fat cheddar or Swiss cheese
⅓ cup Parmesan cheese

METHOD
1. Preheat oven to 350 degrees.
2. In a nonstick saucepan sprayed with nonstick cooking spray, sauté garlic and onion until tender. Add flour and mix well. Add milk and seasonings. Cook until slightly thickened, stirring constantly, about 2 minutes.
3. Alternate layers of potato, cheeses, and sauce in a 2-qt baking dish that has been coated with nonstick cooking spray.
4. Bake for 45 minutes or until bubbly and golden brown. Let stand 20 minutes before serving.

DINNER

66

58g carb

6½ oz beef rib (3 oz meat), grilled and
   basted with
2 Tbsp barbecue sauce
1 Pillsbury buttermilk or country-style biscuit
1 cup steamed green beans flavored with
1 slice Canadian bacon, chopped
3 oz Ore-Ida Zesties fries, baked
¾ cup **Raspberry-Orange Gelatin
Supreme**

Raspberry-Orange Gelatin Supreme

Yield: 6 servings / Serving size: ¾ cup

INGREDIENTS

1 pkg. orange sugar-free gelatin
1 pkg. raspberry sugar-free gelatin
2 cups 100% apple-raspberry juice
2 cups water
1 11-oz can juice-packed mandarin oranges

METHOD

1. Pour gelatin powders into a 2-qt bowl.
2. In a small pan, mix raspberry juice and water and heat
   to boiling.
3. Mix boiling juice mixture and gelatin until gelatin is
   thoroughly dissolved.
4. Chill until thickened but not completely set. Add oranges,
   stirring to spread throughout gelatin. Chill until firm.

67

56g carb

1½ cups **Seafood Casserole**
½ cup asparagus
1 tsp. reduced-fat margarine
Dash lemon juice
Tossed salad
2 Tbsp. reduced-fat salad dressing
1 cup chilled melon balls

Seafood Casserole

Yield: 6 servings / Serving size: 1 cup

INGREDIENTS

1 lb fresh or frozen cooked lump crab meat, thawed
½ lb frozen cooked small shrimp, thawed
1 10-oz package frozen peas, thawed and drained
1½ cups cooked rice
¼ cup chopped green bell pepper
2 Tbsp chopped fresh parsley
1 tsp tarragon
Fresh ground pepper and salt to taste
1 cup low-fat sour cream

METHOD

1. Preheat oven to 350 degrees.
2. Combine all ingredients and place in a 2-qt casserole dish sprayed with nonstick cooking spray.
3. Bake covered for 45 minutes.

DINNER

1 serving **Tofu-Vegetable Stir-Fry**
²/₃ cup cooked brown rice
1 cup tossed salad with
1 Tbsp fat-free Italian dressing
1 piece **Pineapple-Oatmeal Cake**
¹/₂ cup fat-free milk

68

75g carb

Tofu-Vegetable Stir-Fry

Yield: 4 servings / Serving size: 2 cups

INGREDIENTS

¹/₂ lb firm tofu, drained and cubed
2 Tbsp olive oil
1 cup carrots, sliced on the diagonal
2 cups chopped broccoli
1 cup sliced bell pepper
¹/₂ cup chopped onion
2 tsp basil
1¹/₂ Tbsp chopped garlic
1 cup sliced mushrooms
2 Tbsp soy sauce or tamari
¹/₄ cup sesame seeds

METHOD

1. Sauté tofu in oil. Flip cubes once or twice to brown on a few sides, about 5 minutes.
2. Add carrots and mix; then add broccoli, peppers, onions, basil, and garlic. Sauté about 3 minutes, mix, and add mushrooms.
3. Turn off heat, add soy sauce, and cover. Let steam for 1 or 2 minutes. Serve with rice or noodles and top with sesame seeds.

DINNER

Pineapple-Oatmeal Cake

Yield: 9 servings / Serving size: 3-inch square

INGREDIENTS

1½ cups quick-cooking oats
4 Tbsp brown sugar substitute
3 Tbsp fat-free dry milk
4 Tbsp whole-wheat flour
2 tsp baking powder
¼ tsp baking soda
2 tsp cinnamon
2 cups crushed juice-packed pineapple, undrained
2 eggs
1 tsp vanilla
2 Tbsp corn oil

METHOD

1. Preheat oven to 375 degrees.
2. Combine all ingredients in a large bowl. Mix well.
3. Coat a 9-inch-square pan with nonstick cooking spray and pour in mixture. Bake for 25 minutes.

DINNER

2 oz. Italian turkey sausage, grilled
2 wedges **Polenta**
½ cup **Marinara Sauce**
2 Tbsp Parmesan cheese
Spinach and green salad
2 Tbsp reduced-fat salad dressing
1 small nectarine

69

77g carb

Polenta

Yield: 4 servings (8 wedges) / Serving size: 2 wedges

INGREDIENTS
4 cups chicken broth
1⅓ cups polenta or coarse-ground cornmeal
1¼ cups water

METHOD
1. Heat broth just to a boil.
2. Combine polenta and water in large saucepot. Add broth to pot, stirring with a whisk to prevent lumps.
3. Cook uncovered over medium heat 30–45 minutes until very thick, stirring as needed to prevent lumps.
4. Spread into a circle about ½-inch thick on a nonstick cookie sheet. Keep warm in oven for immediate use or cool and keep for future use. When set, cut into 8 wedges. Serve with marinara sauce on top.

DINNER

Marinara Sauce

Yield: 2 servings / Serving size: ½ cup

INGREDIENTS

¼ cup low-sodium chicken broth
1 small onion, diced
1 clove garlic, crushed
¾ cup tomato sauce
1 tsp dry mustard
4 Tbsp lemon juice
½ tsp oregano
½ tsp parsley

METHOD

Simmer all ingredients uncovered for 20 minutes.

70

73g carb

1 **Bean Burger**
1 oz Swiss cheese
1 cup green beans
1 tsp margarine
1 cup tossed salad
1 Tbsp reduced-fat salad dressing
2 **Breakfast in a Cookie**
6 fresh cherries
1 cup fat-free milk

Bean Burgers

Yield: 8 servings / Serving size: 1 burger

INGREDIENTS
1 16-oz can kidney, pinto, or black beans
2 cups cooked brown rice or millet
2 Tbsp ketchup
2 cloves garlic, minced
1 tsp dried oregano
1 tsp dried basil
¼ cup Parmesan cheese
¼ cup finely chopped onions
Salt and pepper to taste (optional)

METHOD
1. Combine all ingredients in a large bowl and mash with a fork or potato masher.
2. Divide mixture into 8 burgers, making patties about ½ inch thick. You may need to wet your hands to keep the mixture from sticking.
3. Coat a nonstick skillet with vegetable spray. Cook burgers over medium heat until browned on both sides, about 7–9 minutes.

Breakfast in a Cookie

Yield: 3½–4 dozen / Serving size: 2 cookies

INGREDIENTS
⅓ cup whole-bran cereal, wheat or oat
½ cup orange juice
¼ cup honey or sugar
¼ cup unsweetened applesauce
1 egg or 2 egg whites
2 tsp vanilla
1 cup whole-wheat pastry flour
1 tsp baking powder
½ tsp baking soda
⅓ cup fat-free dry milk
2 tsp grated orange rind
2 tsp cinnamon
1 tsp nutmeg
1 cup quick-cooking rolled oats
½ cup finely chopped nuts
1 cup raisins

METHOD
1. Preheat oven to 375 degrees.
2. In a small bowl, combine bran and orange juice; set aside.
3. In a large bowl, mix honey and applesauce; add egg and mix.
4. Blend in bran–orange juice mixture and add vanilla.
5. Add remaining ingredients to wet mixture.
6. Drop by level teaspoonful onto cookie sheets coated with nonstick cooking spray, about 2 inches apart, and bake for 10–12 minutes or until golden brown.

DINNER

1 serving **Chicken Casserole**
4 pecan halves
Tossed salad with

71

53g carb   1 oz shredded cheddar cheese
2 Tbsp reduced-fat salad dressing
1 slice **Chocolate Angel Food Cake** (see
page 141)
1 cup raspberries, fresh or frozen,
unsweetened

Chicken Casserole

Yield: 4 servings / Serving size: 1 cup

INGREDIENTS

1 Tbsp reduced-fat margarine
1 Tbsp oat flour
½ tsp salt (optional)
¾ cup fat-free milk
1 cup sliced mushrooms

2 tsp Parmesan cheese
⅔ cup cubed cooked chicken
⅔ cup broccoli florets
3 Tbsp chopped onion
2 Tbsp toasted oats

METHOD

1. Preheat oven to 350 degrees.
2. Prepare white sauce by melting margarine in medium saucepan. Add oat flour and stir until all flour is coated evenly. Stir in salt. Slowly add milk, stirring constantly. Heat sauce to boiling, stirring frequently. Cook 1 minute to thicken.
3. Add mushrooms. Stir and cook 1 minute. Remove from heat and add cheese. Mix well.
4. In medium mixing bowl, combine chicken, broccoli, and onion. Stir in sauce and mix well to coat all ingredients.
5. Pour into 1-qt casserole. Top with oats. Bake for 30 minutes.

1 serving **Hearty Onion-Garlic Soup**
2 Tbsp Parmesan cheese
1 whole-wheat roll
½ Tbsp reduced-calorie margarine
¼ cup fresh fruit salad
1 cup fat-free milk

72

77g carb

Hearty Onion-Garlic Soup

Yield: 4 servings / Serving size: 1½ cups

INGREDIENTS
2 cups sliced onions
1 cup sliced green pepper
2 Tbsp olive oil
20 garlic cloves, sliced
3 cups canned diced tomatoes
2 cups vegetable broth
4 slices dark or whole-wheat bread, cut in ¼-inch cubes
   and toasted
Black pepper to taste

METHOD
1. In large saucepan, sauté onions and pepper in oil until
   soft and golden.
2. Add garlic and tomatoes. Reduce heat, cover pan, and
   simmer for 30 minutes.
3. Add broth; heat to a boil.
4. Add bread cubes and pepper just before serving.

DINNER

1 serving **Spinach-Stuffed Chicken Breasts**

1 cup steamed new potatoes

Lettuce with
½ cup grapefruit sections,
1 Tbsp French dressing, and
1 Tbsp slivered almonds

73

57g carb

Spinach-Stuffed Chicken Breasts

Yield: 4 servings / Serving size: ½ breast

INGREDIENTS

½ 10-oz pkg. frozen chopped spinach, defrosted and
   drained
¼ cup low-fat ricotta cheese
¼ cup shredded part-skim mozzarella cheese
¼ tsp tarragon
4 boneless chicken breast halves, (leave skin intact)
½ tsp reduced-fat margarine, melted

METHOD

1. Preheat oven to 350 degrees.
2. Combine spinach, cheeses, and seasonings.
3. Lift up skin of each chicken breast and divide mixture
   evenly among them. Be careful not to tear skins.
   Smooth skin over stuffing; tuck skin edges underneath
   to form a neat package.
4. Brush chicken with melted margarine. Place in 2-qt
   baking dish.
5. Bake uncovered for 45–50 minutes.
6. Remove skin before serving.

Tortellini Primavera
74
73g carb

1 cup tossed green salad
1 Tbsp fat-free dressing
4 whole-grain crackers
½ cup fat-free milk

Tortellini Primavera

Yield: 1 serving

INGREDIENTS
½ cup fresh or frozen cheese tortellini
⅓ cup each sliced or chopped broccoli, mushrooms,
zucchini, and asparagus
1 tsp minced garlic
1 tsp olive oil
½ cup fat-free milk
1 tsp cornstarch
Pinch nutmeg
Freshly ground pepper
1 Tbsp chopped fresh parsley
2 Tbsp sliced green onion
2 Tbsp Parmesan cheese

METHOD
1. Boil water and cook tortellini according to package directions while proceeding with the vegetables.
2. Sauté vegetables and garlic in nonstick skillet with oil on medium-high heat for about 1 minute. Reduce heat and cover for 1–2 more minutes until tender-crisp.
3. Combine milk and cornstarch and add it to the vegetables. Stir constantly until thickened.
4. Add nutmeg and pepper to taste. Toss together with tortellini, parsley, and onion. Sprinkle with Parmesan cheese.

DINNER

1 serving **Dahl**
½ cup cooked carrots
½ cup cooked green beans
9 dry-roasted almonds
Café Mocha:
   ½ cup strong coffee
   ½ cup scalded fat-free milk, whipped
   ½ tsp. cocoa
   Sugar substitute to taste

75

77g carb

Mix coffee and milk in tall mug and sprinkle with sweetener and cocoa.

Dahl

Yield: 2 servings / Serving size: ½ recipe

INGREDIENTS

1 cup lentils
2 tsp canola oil
1 medium onion, chopped
2 cloves garlic, chopped
2 tsp coriander

½ tsp cayenne pepper
¼ tsp turmeric
½ tsp ginger
½ tsp cumin
1 cup water

METHOD

1. Rinse and soak lentils for 1 hour.
2. Heat oil in medium skillet and sauté onion and garlic for 3–4 minutes. Add spices and sauté for 2 minutes.
3. Add drained lentils and sauté 5 minutes. Add water, cover and simmer about 1 hour. Add more water if necessary to keep lentils from sticking to the pan, but most of the water should be absorbed after 1 hour.

DINNER

Snacks

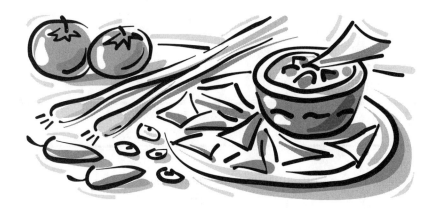

Each 60-calorie snack includes
1 starch serving OR
1 fruit serving OR
2 vegetable servings

Each 125-calorie snack includes
1 starch serving and
1 fat serving OR
1 meat substitute serving and
1 fruit serving

Each 170-calorie snack includes
1 starch serving and
1 fat-free milk serving OR
2 starch servings OR
1 starch serving and
1 meat serving

60-Calorie Snacks

½ cup strawberries
4 animal crackers

13g carb

1 frozen fruit juice bar

19g carb

2 cups mixed carrot, squash, and bell
   pepper sticks with
1 Tbsp reduced-fat Ranch dressing

17g carb

15 baked tortilla chips with
¼ cup salsa

21g carb

Grapefruit Cooler:
    8 oz sugar-free ginger ale and
    ½ cup grapefruit juice

11g carb

SNACKS

Macedonia Fruit Cup

Yield: 10 servings / Serving size: ½ cup

INGREDIENTS

¾ cup orange juice
4 tsp lemon juice
15 seedless grapes
12 cherries, pitted
1 medium apple, peeled and thinly sliced
1 medium pear, peeled and thinly sliced
1 medium banana, peeled and thinly sliced
1 small plum, thinly sliced
1 medium peach, thinly sliced
¼ cup honeydew melon, cubed
¾ cup strawberries, stemmed and halved

METHOD

1. Pour orange and lemon juice into a large serving bowl.
   Add grapes and cherries.
2. Add other fruits to the bowl immediately after cutting to
   prevent discoloration. Toss gently.
3. Serve chilled.

SNACKS

½ cup **Fruit Punch**

7

13g carb

Fruit Punch

Yield: 12 servings / Serving size: ½ cup

INGREDIENTS

2 cups unsweetened pineapple juice, chilled
2 cups low-calorie cranberry juice cocktail, chilled
¾ cup orange juice, chilled
¾ cup club soda, chilled
Ice cubes
Lime and orange slices

METHOD

Combine all ingredients in a punch bowl just before serving.

17 **Frosty Grapes**

8

12g carb

Frosty Grapes

Yield: 4 servings / Serving size: about 17 grapes

INGREDIENTS

1 lb seedless grapes
1 0.4-oz pkg. sugar-free lime gelatin

METHOD

1. Divide grapes into small bunches. Rinse and drain.
2. Put gelatin powder in a container with a lid that can be frozen. Add grapes and shake to coat. Shake off excess powder from grape bunches.
3. Put lid on container and freeze. Serve frozen.

½ frozen banana on a stick dipped in
2 Tbsp **Chocolate-Flavored Syrup**

9

19g carb

Chocolate-Flavored Syrup

Yield: 15 servings / Serving size: 2 Tbsp

INGREDIENTS

½ cup dry cocoa, firmly packed
1½ cups cold water
¼ tsp salt
Sugar substitute to substitute for ½ cup sugar
2½ tsp vanilla

METHOD

1. Mix cocoa, water, and salt in a heavy saucepan until smooth. Bring to a boil and simmer gently, stirring constantly, for 3 minutes.
2. Remove from heat and let cool 10 minutes.
3. Add sugar substitute and vanilla and mix well.
4. Store refrigerated in a jar. Stir well in jar before measuring to use.

SNACKS

½ cup **Strawberry Whip**

10

17g carb

Strawberry Whip

Yield: 4 servings / Serving size: ¾ cup

INGREDIENTS
3-oz pkg sugar-free gelatin
1 cup fat-free plain yogurt
1 cup sliced strawberries

METHOD
1. Prepare gelatin according to instructions on package.
2. Beat hardened gelatin with rotary beater until frothy. Add yogurt and beat gently until mixed.
3. Stir strawberries into gelatin-yogurt mixture.
4. Freeze 10 minutes, then serve.

125-Calorie Snacks

11

25g carb

1 cup tomato soup
4 saltine crackers

12

19g carb

1 cup popcorn
¼ oz pretzels
¼ cup Cheerios
20 small peanuts

Mix together for party or trail mix.

13

23g carb

½ slice angel food cake topped with
½ cup sliced strawberries and
2 Tbsp whipped topping

SNACKS

1 slice French bread, broiled with
1 tsp margarine
1 Tbsp Parmesan cheese
Basil

13g carb

4 RyKrisp crackers, divided into 12 sections,
   topped with
Cheese Spread:
   1½ Tbsp reduced-fat cream cheese
   1 tsp dried onion flakes and
Cucumber, red pepper, and green onion
   slices

20g carb

No-Fat Steak Fries

25g carb

Slice a leftover baked potato with skin into wedges and place on nonstick cookie sheet. Spray with butter-flavored nonstick cooking spray and broil until golden.

¼ cup low-fat cottage cheese (4.5%)
½ cup pineapple chunks packed in juice

21g carb

½ cup water-packed fruit cocktail
½ cup fat-free artificially sweetened yogurt

27g carb

1 oz string cheese
1 small apple

17g carb

⅓ cup **Black Bean Dip** with
Vegetable chips (sliced raw carrots,
cauliflower, broccoli, and celery)

20

21g carb

Black Bean Dip

Yield: 2 cups / Serving size: ⅓ cup

INGREDIENTS

1 15-oz can black beans, drained
1 small onion, chopped
1 small green pepper, chopped
1 clove garlic, chopped
1½ Tbsp red wine vinegar
1½ Tbsp olive oil
½ tsp sugar
Salt, pepper, and hot sauce to taste

METHOD

1. Combine all ingredients in a food processor.
2. Process, pushing off and on until beans are coarsely mashed.
3. Season to taste.

170-Calorie Snacks

½ Meat Sandwich:
1 slice bread
1 oz turkey or ham
1 tsp margarine or mayonnaise

12g carb

1 hard-boiled egg
2 slices lite wheat bread
1 tsp reduced-fat mayonnaise

19g carb

1 Mini Pizza:
½ English muffin
1 Tbsp pizza sauce
1 oz part-skim mozzarella cheese
1 cup tossed salad
1 Tbsp reduced-fat salad dressing

19g carb

Heat topped muffin until cheese melts.

½ bagel with
1 Tbsp peanut butter

22g carb

SNACKS

2 Baked Potato Skins

28g carb

Split baked potato in half and scoop out all but ⅛–¼ inch of potato flesh; sprinkle with 1 oz shredded part-skim mozzarella cheese and paprika, then bake in 450-degree oven or broil until cheese melts and bubbles.

24 Oyster Hors d'Oeuvres

17g carb

Mix 24 oyster crackers with 1 Tbsp melted margarine. Sprinkle with a powdered reduced-calorie Ranch salad dressing. Broil until browned.

2 Graham Pudding Sandwiches
(see page 29)

27g carb

SNACKS

1 **Vanilla Milkshake**

Vanilla Milkshake

Yield: 1 serving / Serving size: 1¼ cups

INGREDIENTS
½ cup sugar-free, fat-free frozen yogurt
1 cup fat-free milk
½ tsp vanilla

METHOD
Blend all ingredients together in blender.

1 Peachy Whole-Grain Cookie
1 cup fat-free or low-fat (1%) milk

29

23g carb

Peachy Whole-Grain Cookie

Yield: 30 cookies / Serving size: 1 cookie

INGREDIENTS
1 egg white
½ tsp almond extract
⅓ cup margarine, softened
6 Tbsp sugar
6 Tbsp packed brown sugar
¾ cup whole-wheat flour
½ tsp salt
1 tsp baking powder
1¼ cups quick-cooking oats
¾ cup diced peaches
¼ cup chopped dates

METHOD
1. Preheat oven to 350 degrees.
2. Beat egg white with extract, margarine, and sugars in mixing bowl.
3. Combine flour, salt, and baking powder. Add to egg mixture and mix well with electric mixer.
4. Stir in oats, peaches, and dates. Drop by rounded (not heaping) tablespoonfuls onto nonstick cookie sheet.
5. Bake for 15 minutes or until golden.

10 Tortilla Chips
½ cup **Oklahoma Bean Salad**

30

32g carb

Cut fresh or frozen corn tortillas into 6 wedges and place on a baking sheet. Bake for 5 minutes in a preheated 500-degree oven. Cool and store in airtight container.

Oklahoma Bean Salad

Yield: 5 cups / Serving size: ½ cup

INGREDIENTS
1 15-oz can black-eyed peas, rinsed and drained
1 15-oz can kidney beans, rinsed and drained
1 15-oz can hominy, rinsed and drained
1 cup chopped tomato
2 Tbsp chopped green onion
1 Tbsp chopped garlic
1 jalapeno pepper, finely chopped (optional)
¾ cup fat-free Italian dressing
1 Tbsp lime juice
2 tsp Italian seasoning
¼ cup chopped cilantro (optional)

METHOD
Mix all ingredients and refrigerate for at least 2 hours before serving to let flavors blend.

SNACKS

Nutritional Analyses

Analyses are in the order the recipes appear in the book.

Sugar-Free Blueberry Muffins

12 servings
Serving size: 1 muffin
Exchanges
1 Starch
1 Fat
Calories 137
   Calories from Fat 52
Total Fat 6 g
   Saturated Fat 0 g
Cholesterol 36 mg
Sodium 103 mg
Total carbohydrate 18 g
   Dietary Fiber 1 g
   Sugars 3 g
Protein 3 g

Ricotta Cheese Spread

1 serving
Serving size: ¼ cup
Exchanges
1 Medium-Fat Meat
Calories 89
   Calories from Fat 44
Total Fat 5 g
   Saturated Fat 3 g
Cholesterol 19 mg
Sodium 76 mg
Total carbohydrate 4 g
   Dietary Fiber 0 g
   Sugars 2 g
Protein 7 g

Easy Spud Breakfast

2 servings
Serving size: ½ recipe
Exchanges
1½ Starch

1 Medium-Fat Meat
Calories 189
   Calories from Fat 45
Total Fat 5 g
   Saturated Fat 2 g
Cholesterol 119 mg
Sodium 287 mg
Total Carbohydrate 26 g
   Dietary Fiber 3 g
   Sugars 4 g
Protein 11 g

Scones

16 servings
Serving size: ¹⁄₁₆th recipe
Exchanges
1 Starch
Calories 76
   Calories from Fat 12
Total Fat 1 g
   Saturated Fat 0 g
Cholesterol 0 mg
Sodium 94 mg
Total Carbohydrate 14 g
   Dietary Fiber 1 g
   Sugars 2 g
Protein 2 g

Graham Pudding Sandwiches

32 servings
Serving size: 1 sandwich
Exchanges
1 Starch
½ Fat
Calories 94
   Calories from Fat 31
Total Fat 3 g
   Saturated Fat 1 g

Cholesterol 0 mg
Sodium 122 mg
Total Carbohydrate 13 g
  Dietary Fiber 1 g
  Sugars 4 g
Protein 3 g

Breakfast Blender Drink
1 serving
Serving size: 1 serving
Exchanges
1 Starch
1 Fruit
1 Fat-Free Milk
Calories 228
  Calories from Fat 26
Total Fat 3 g
  Saturated Fat 0 g
Cholesterol 4 mg
Sodium 128 mg
Total Carbohydrate 38 g
  Dietary Fiber 4 g
  Sugars 24 g
Protein 15 g

Crunchy Granola
16 servings
Serving size: 1/3 cup
Exchanges
1 1/2 Carbohydrate
2 Fat
Calories 198
  Calories from Fat 90
Total Fat 10 g
  Saturated Fat 2 g
Cholesterol 0 mg
Sodium 3 mg
Total Carbohydrate 24 g
  Dietary Fiber 4 g
  Sugars 8 g
Protein 5 g

Cheesy Grits
2 servings
Serving size: 1 cup
Exchanges
2 Starch
2 Medium-Fat Meat
1 Fat
Calories 342
  Calories from Fat 136
Total Fat 15 g
  Saturated Fat 7 g
Cholesterol 137 mg
Sodium 431 mg
Total Carbohydrate 32 g
  Dietary Fiber 2 g
  Sugars 3 g
Protein 21 g

Apple-Raisin Muffins
12 servings
Serving size: 1 muffin
Exchanges
1 Starch
1/2 Fruit
1/2 Fat
Calories 145
  Calories from Fat 38
Total Fat 4 g
  Saturated Fat 0 g
Cholesterol 18 mg
Sodium 151 mg
Total Carbohydrate 24 g
  Dietary Fiber 1 g
  Sugars 7 g
Protein 3 g

Creamed Chipped Beef over Toast
2 servings
Serving size: 1/2 recipe
Exchanges
1 Starch
1 Very Lean Meat

½ Fat-Free Milk
1 Fat
Calories 207
Calories from Fat 57
Total Fat 6 g
Saturated Fat 1 g
Cholesterol 14 mg
Sodium 1237 mg
Total Carbohydrate 22 g
Dietary Fiber 2 g
Sugars 7 g
Protein 16 g

Angel Biscuits
36 servings
Serving size: 1 biscuit
Exchanges
1 Starch
1 Fat
Calories 122
Calories from Fat 54
Total Fat 6 g
Saturated Fat 1 g
Cholesterol 0 mg
Sodium 209 mg
Total Carbohydrate 15 g
Dietary Fiber 1 g
Sugars 2 g
Protein 3 g

Spanish Omelet
4 servings
Serving size: ¼th recipe
Exchanges
1 Very Lean Meat
1 Vegetable
Calories 71
Calories from Fat 4
Total Fat 0 g
Saturated Fat 0 g
Cholesterol 1 mg
Sodium 338 mg
Total Carbohydrate 7 g

Dietary Fiber 2 g
Sugars 4 g
Protein 9 g

Grapefruit Grand
1 serving
Serving size: 1 serving
Exchanges
1 Fruit
Calories 57
Calories from Fat 2
Total Fat 0 g
Saturated Fat 0 g
Cholesterol 0 mg
Sodium 0 mg
Total Carbohydrate 14 g
Dietary Fiber 2 g
Sugars 11 g
Protein 1 g

Broccoli Quiche
6 servings
Serving size: ⅙th recipe
Exchanges
1 Starch
1 Medium-Fat Meat
1 Fat
Calories 192
Calories from Fat 96
Total Fat 11 g
Saturated Fat 5 g
Cholesterol 127 mg
Sodium 317 mg
Total Carbohydrate 13 g
Dietary Fiber 2 g
Sugars 5 g
Protein 12 g

Fluffy High-Fiber, Low-Fat Pancakes
4 servings
Serving size: 2 pancakes
Exchanges

1 ½ Starch
Calories 132
   Calories from Fat 28
Total Fat 3 g
   Saturated Fat 1 g
Cholesterol 55 mg
Sodium 462 mg
Total Carbohydrate 23 g
   Dietary Fiber 7 g
   Sugars 4 g
Protein 8 g

Tofu Garden Quiche

8 servings
Serving size: ⅛th recipe
Exchanges
1 Lean Meat
1 Vegetable
Calories 78
   Calories from Fat 38
Total Fat 4 g
   Saturated Fat 1 g
Cholesterol 53 mg
Sodium 38 mg
Total Carbohydrate 5 g
   Dietary Fiber 1 g
   Sugars 3 g
Protein 6 g

Peanut Butter and Jelly Muffin

12 servings
Serving size: 1 muffin
Exchanges
2 Starch
1 ½ Fat
Calories 216
   Calories from Fat 81
Total Fat 9 g
   Saturated Fat 2 g
Cholesterol 19 mg
Sodium 183 mg
Total Carbohydrate 28 g

Dietary Fiber 2 g
Sugars 9 g
Protein 7 g

Iowa Corn Pancakes

8 servings
Serving size: 2 pancakes
Exchanges
1 Starch
Calories 79
   Calories from Fat 8
Total Fat 1 g
   Saturated Fat 0 g
Cholesterol 1 mg
Sodium 222 mg
Total Carbohydrate 15 g
   Dietary Fiber 2 g
   Sugars 2 g
Protein 4 g

Sweet Potato-Raisin Cookies

12 servings
Serving size: 2 cookies
Exchanges
2 Carbohydrate
1 Fat
Calories 186
   Calories from Fat 57
Total Fat 6 g
   Saturated Fat 3 g
Cholesterol 28 mg
Sodium 256 mg
Total Carbohydrate 31 g
   Dietary Fiber 4 g
   Sugars 12 g
Protein 5 g

Baked Rice Pudding

4 servings
Serving size: ⅔ cup
Exchanges
2 Starch

Calories 173
  Calories from Fat 25
Total Fat 3 g
  Saturated Fat 1 g
Cholesterol 108 mg
Sodium 134 mg
Total Carbohydrate 29 g
  Dietary Fiber 0 g
  Sugars 6 g
Protein 7 g

Low Country Grits and Sausage

2 servings
Serving size: ½ recipe
Exchanges
2½ Starch
1 Medium-Fat Meat
Calories 285
  Calories from Fat 68
Total Fat 8 g
  Saturated Fat 3 g
Cholesterol 231 mg
Sodium 316 mg
Total Carbohydrate 35 g
  Dietary Fiber 0 g
  Sugars 4 g
Protein 18 g

Johnnycake

12 servings
Serving size: 1 slice
Exchanges
1½ Starch
½ Fat
Calories 135
  Calories from Fat 28
Total Fat 3 g
  Saturated Fat 0 g
Cholesterol 1 mg
Sodium 458 mg
Total Carbohydrate 22 g
  Dietary Fiber 2 g

Sugars 4 g
Protein 4 g

Granola Pancakes

6 servings
Serving size: 3 pancakes
Exchanges
3 Starch
½ Fat
Calories 254
  Calories from Fat 34
Total Fat 4 g
  Saturated Fat 1 g
Cholesterol 72 mg
Sodium 196 mg
Total Carbohydrate 46 g
  Dietary Fiber 6 g
  Sugars 12 g
Protein 12 g

Atomic Muffins

24 servings
Serving size: 1 muffin
Exchanges
1 Starch
1 Lean Meat
1½ Fat
Calories 202
  Calories from Fat 114
Total Fat 13 g
  Saturated Fat 2 g
Cholesterol 19 mg
Sodium 83 mg
Total Carbohydrate 18 g
  Dietary Fiber 3 g
  Sugars 10 g
Protein 6 g

Oatmeal–Wheatena Porridge with Bananas and Walnuts

1 serving
Serving size: 1 recipe

Exchanges
2½ Starch
1 Fruit
1 Fat
Calories 288
   Calories from Fat 60
Total Fat 7 g
   Saturated Fat 0 g
Cholesterol 0 mg
Sodium 6 mg
Total Carbohydrate 50 g
   Dietary Fiber 7 g
   Sugars 13 g
Protein 8 g

Whole-Wheat Currant Scones
16 servings
Serving size: 1 scone
Exchanges
1½ Starch
½ Fat
Calories 130
   Calories from Fat 26
Total Fat 3 g
   Saturated Fat 1 g
Cholesterol 27 mg
Sodium 209 mg
Total Carbohydrate 22 g
   Dietary Fiber 2 g
   Sugars 5 g
Protein 5 g

French Dressing
6 servings
Serving size: 2 Tbsp.
Free food
Calories 6
   Calories from Fat 0
Total Fat 0 g
   Saturated Fat 0 g
Cholesterol 0 mg
Sodium 268 mg

Total Carbohydrate 2 g
   Dietary Fiber 0 g
   Sugars 1 g
Protein 0 g

Whole-Wheat Pizza
8 servings
Serving size: 1 slice
Exchanges
2 Starch
1 Medium-Fat Meat
Calories 233
   Calories from Fat 60
Total Fat 7 g
   Saturated Fat 3 g
Cholesterol 14 mg
Sodium 391 mg
Total Carbohydrate 34 g
   Dietary Fiber 5 g
   Sugars 4 g
Protein 12 g

Noodle Supreme Salad
2 servings
Serving size: 1 cup
Exchanges
2 Starch
1 Very Lean Meat
Calories 179
   Calories from Fat 18
Total Fat 2 g
   Saturated Fat 1 g
Cholesterol 35 mg
Sodium 206 mg
Total Carbohydrate 27 g
   Dietary Fiber 3 g
   Sugars 3 g
Protein 13 g

Black Bean Soup
4 servings
Serving size: 1 cup
Exchanges

2½ Starch
1 Very Lean Meat
Calories 223
  Calories from Fat 35
Total Fat 4 g
  Saturated Fat 1 g
Cholesterol 0 mg
Sodium 5 mg
Total Carbohydrate 36 g
  Dietary Fiber 12 g
  Sugars 7 g
Protein 12 g

Sloppy Joes
6 servings
Serving size: 1/2 cup
Exchanges
2 Medium-Fat Meat
1 Vegetable
Calories 167
  Calories from Fat 90
Total Fat 10 g
  Saturated Fat 4 g
Cholesterol 47 mg
Sodium 311 mg
Total Carbohydrate 5 g
  Dietary Fiber 1 g
  Sugars 3 g
Protein 14 g

English Muffin Pizza Melt
6 servings
Serving size: ⅙th recipe
Exchanges
1 Starch
2 Medium-Fat Meat
Calories 243
  Calories from Fat 102
Total Fat 11 g
  Saturated Fat 4 g
Cholesterol 49 mg
Sodium 460 mg

Total Carbohydrate 17 g
  Dietary Fiber 1 g
  Sugars 3 g
Protein 17 g

Tortilla Ranch Style
1 serving
Serving size: 1 tortilla
Exchanges
2½ Starch
2 Medium-Fat Meat
1 Vegetable
1 Fat
Calories 421
  Calories from Fat 163
Total Fat 18 g
  Saturated Fat 7 g
Cholesterol 57 mg
Sodium 819 mg
Total Carbohydrate 42 g
  Dietary Fiber 4 g
  Sugars 6 g
Protein 20 g

Submarine Sandwich
4 servings
Serving size: 1 sandwich
Exchanges
2 Starch
2 Very Lean Meat
1 Vegetable
½ Fat
Calories 267
  Calories from Fat 43
Total Fat 5 g
  Saturated Fat 2 g
Cholesterol 38 mg
Sodium 666 mg
Total Carbohydrate 34 g
  Dietary Fiber 2 g
  Sugars 3 g
Protein 22 g

Minestrone
5 servings
Serving size: 1 cup
Exchanges
2 Carbohydrate
1 Fat
Calories 203
　Calories from Fat 33
Total Fat 4 g
　Saturated Fat 1 g
Cholesterol 6 mg
Sodium 747 mg
Total Carbohydrate 32 g
　Dietary Fiber 7 g
　Sugars 8 g
Protein 13 g

Spicy Black-Eyed Peas
4 servings
Serving size: 1¼ cups
Exchanges
1 Starch
2 Vegetable
Calories 130
　Calories from Fat 9
Total Fat 1 g
　Saturated Fat 0 g
Cholesterol 0 mg
Sodium 775 mg
Total Carbohydrate 26 g
　Dietary Fiber 5 g
　Sugars 8 g
Protein 7 g

Crunchy Tuna Cheese Melt
1 serving
Serving size: 1 serving
Exchanges
2 Starch
3 Lean Meat
1 Vegetable
½ Fat

Calories 377
　Calories from Fat 105
Total Fat 12 g
　Saturated Fat 5 g
Cholesterol 47 mg
Sodium 748 mg
Total Carbohydrate 35 g
　Dietary Fiber 5 g
　Sugars 8 g
Protein 34 g

Fast Corn Chowder
4 servings
Serving size: 1 cup
Exchanges
2½ Carbohydrate
½ Fat
Calories 218
　Calories from Fat 41
Total Fat 5 g
　Saturated Fat 1 g
Cholesterol 0 mg
Sodium 698 mg
Total Carbohydrate 37 g
　Dietary Fiber 2 g
　Sugars 19 g
Protein 10 g

Veggie Pizza
2 servings
Serving size: ½ recipe
Exchanges
2 Starch
1 Medium-Fat Meat
2 Vegetable
1 Fat
Calories 330
　Calories from Fat 99
Total Fat 11 g
　Saturated Fat 4 g
Cholesterol 16 mg
Sodium 1163 mg
Total Carbohydrate 41 g

Dietary Fiber 2 g
Sugars 6 g
Protein 16 g

Light Spinach Salad
2 servings
Serving size: ½ recipe
Exchanges
3 Medium-Fat Meat
2 Vegetable
½ Fruit
Calories 302
Calories from Fat 135
Total Fat 15 g
Saturated Fat 7 g
Cholesterol 78 mg
Sodium 422 mg
Total Carbohydrate 19 g
Dietary Fiber 5 g
Sugars 13 g
Protein 28 g

Gazpacho
4 servings
Serving size: 1 cup
Exchanges
3 Vegetable
1 Fat
Calories 116
Calories from Fat 60
Total Fat 7 g
Saturated Fat 1 g
Cholesterol 0 mg
Sodium 416 mg
Total Carbohydrate 14 g
Dietary Fiber 3 g
Sugars 8 g
Protein 2 g

Broiled Open-Faced Vegetarian Sandwich
1 serving
Serving size: 1 sandwich

Exchanges
3 Starch
2 Medium-Fat Meat
2 Vegetable
1 Fat
Calories 486
Calories from Fat 168
Total Fat 9 g
Saturated Fat 7 g
Cholesterol 32 mg
Sodium 800 mg
Total Carbohydrate 59 g
Dietary Fiber 6 g
Sugars 13 g
Protein 23 g

Spicy Turkey Loaf
8 servings
Serving size: ⅛th recipe
Exchanges
1 Starch
3 Very Lean Meat
Calories 170
Calories from Fat 28
Total Fat 3 g
Saturated Fat 1 g
Cholesterol 56 mg
Sodium 277 mg
Total Carbohydrate 12 g
Dietary Fiber 0 g
Sugars 4 g
Protein 22 g

Pizza Muffins
6 servings
Serving size: 2 muffins
Exchanges
2 Starch
½ Fat
Calories 190
Calories from Fat 40
Total Fat 4 g
Saturated Fat 2 g

Cholesterol 42 mg
Sodium 555 mg
Total Carbohydrate 29 g
  Dietary Fiber 5 g
  Sugars 5 g
Protein 11 g

Fiesta Rice
4 servings
Serving size: 1 cup
Exchanges
2½ Starch
1 Lean Meat
Calories 238
  Calories from Fat 34
Total Fat 4 g
  Saturated Fat 1 g
Cholesterol 8 mg
Sodium 367 mg
Total Carbohydrate 34 g
  Dietary Fiber 3 g
  Sugars 6 g
Protein 17 g

Turkey-Squash Casserole
6 servings
Serving size: ⅙th recipe
Exchanges
2 Starch
2 Very Lean Meat
1 Vegetable
1 Fat
Calories 298
  Calories from Fat 47
Total Fat 5 g
  Saturated Fat 1 g
Cholesterol 73 mg
Sodium 617 mg
Total Carbohydrate 37 g
  Dietary Fiber 5 g
  Sugars 9 g
Protein 22 g

Pan-Broiled Shrimp
2 servings
Serving size: ½ recipe
Exchanges
2 Very Lean Meat
½ Fat
Calories 89
  Calories from Fat 23
Total Fat 3 g
  Saturated Fat 0 g
Cholesterol 116 mg
Sodium 156 mg
Total Carbohydrate 3 g
  Dietary Fiber 1 g
  Sugars 2 g
Protein 13 g

Spanish Garbanzo Beans
2 servings
Serving size: 1 cup
Exchanges
2 Starch
3 Vegetable
2½ Fat
Calories 345
  Calories from Fat 137
Total Fat 15 g
  Saturated Fat 3 g
Cholesterol 0 mg
Sodium 694 mg
Total Carbohydrate 44 g
  Dietary Fiber 11 g
  Sugars 15 g
Protein 12 g

Schinkennudelin
1 serving
Serving size: 1 serving
Exchanges
1½ Starch
2 Lean Meat
1 Fat
Calories 275

Calories from Fat 124
Total Fat 14 g
  Saturated Fat 3 g
Cholesterol 255 mg
Sodium 520 mg
Total Carbohydrate 21 g
  Dietary Fiber 1 g
  Sugars 2 g
Protein 17 g

Lentil-Veggie Soup
4 servings
Serving size: 1½ cups
Exchanges
Starch 3.0
2 Very Lean Meat
3 Vegetable
1 Fat
Calories 425
  Calories from Fat 62
Total Fat 7 g
  Saturated Fat 0 g
Cholesterol 24 mg
Sodium 524 mg
Total Carbohydrate 63 g
  Dietary Fiber 23 g
  Sugars 12 g
Protein 32 g

Seven-Layer Salad
2 servings
Serving size: ½ recipe
Exchanges
1 Starch
3 Medium-Fat Meat
1 Vegetable
½ Fat
Calories 345
  Calories from Fat 175
Total Fat 19 g
  Saturated Fat 7 g
Cholesterol 244 mg
Sodium 648 mg

Total Carbohydrate 22 g
  Dietary Fiber 7 g
  Sugars 10 g
Protein 22 g

Caesar Salad
3 servings
Serving size: ⅓ recipe
Exchanges
1½ Starch
1 Medium-Fat Meat
1 Vegetable
2½ Fat
Calories 335
  Calories from Fat 176
Total Fat 20 g
  Saturated Fat 6 g
Cholesterol 97 mg
Sodium 1057 mg
Total Carbohydrate 26 g
  Dietary Fiber 1 g
  Sugars 7 g
Protein 16 g

Pintos and Potatoes
6 servings
Serving size: ⅙th recipe
Exchanges
2 Starch
1 Very Lean Meat
½ Fat
Calories 194
  Calories from Fat 41
Total Fat 5 g
  Saturated Fat 1 g
Cholesterol 0 mg
Sodium 199 mg
Total Carbohydrate 31 g
  Dietary Fiber 9 g
  Sugars 3 g
Protein 9 g

Mastokhiar

2 servings
Serving size: 1 cup
Exchanges
1 Vegetable
1 Fruit
1 Reduced-Fat Milk
Calories 183
  Calories from Fat 28
Total Fat 3 g
  Saturated Fat 2 g
Cholesterol 15 mg
Sodium 273 mg
Total Carbohydrate 31 g
  Dietary Fiber 2 g
  Sugars 27 g
Protein 11 g

Shrimp and Pea Salad

4 servings
Serving size: ¼th recipe
Exchanges
1 Starch
2 Very Lean Meat
Calories 162
  Calories from Fat 12
Total Fat 1 g
  Saturated Fat 0 g
Cholesterol 112 mg
Sodium 289 mg
Total Carbohydrate 18 g
  Dietary Fiber 6 g
  Sugars 9 g
Protein 19 g

Low-Fat Lemon Cheesecake

16 servings
Serving size: 1 slice
Exchanges
1 Carbohydrate

Calories 101
  Calories from Fat 2
Total Fat 0 g
  Saturated Fat 0 g
Cholesterol 4 mg
Sodium 196 mg
Total Carbohydrate 18 g
  Dietary Fiber 0 g
  Sugars 15 g
Protein 7 g

Southwestern Veggie Soup

4 servings
Serving size: 1 cup
Exchanges
2 Starch
1 Medium-Fat Meat
Calories 230
  Calories from Fat 58
Total Fat 6 g
  Saturated Fat 3 g
Cholesterol 16 mg
Sodium 453 mg
Total Carbohydrate 33 g
  Dietary Fiber 6 g
  Sugars 6 g
Protein 13 g

Hummus with Red Pepper

6 servings
Serving size: ⅓ cup
Exchanges
1 Starch
1 Very Lean Meat
1 Fat
Calories 145
  Calories from Fat 62
Total Fat 7 g
  Saturated Fat 1 g
Cholesterol 0 mg
Sodium 55 mg

Total Carbohydrate 17 g
  Dietary Fiber 5 g
  Sugars 4 g
Protein 6 g

Cucumbers with Dill Dressing

3 servings
Serving size: ¾ cup
Exchanges
2 Vegetable
1 Fat
Calories 80
  Calories from Fat 45
Total Fat 5 g
  Saturated Fat 0 g
Cholesterol 0 mg
Sodium 6 mg
Total Carbohydrate 9 g
  Dietary Fiber 2 g
  Sugars 6 g
Protein 1 g

Bean Salad

6 servings
Serving size: 1 cup
Exchanges
1 Starch
1 Vegetable
½ Fat
Calories 126
  Calories from Fat 41
Total Fat 5 g
  Saturated Fat 1 g
Cholesterol 0 mg
Sodium 9 mg
Total Carbohydrate 18 g
  Dietary Fiber 5 g
  Sugars 4 g
Protein 5 g

Whole-Grain Muffin

8 servings
Serving size: 1 muffin
Exchanges
1 Starch
½ Fat
Calories 95
  Calories from Fat 26
Total Fat 3 g
  Saturated Fat 0 g
Cholesterol 28 mg
Sodium 378 mg
Total Carbohydrate 14 g
  Dietary Fiber 2 g
  Sugars 3 g
Protein 4 g

Rigatoni Salad

8 servings
Serving size: ½ cup
Exchanges
1½ Starch
1 Vegetable
Calories 132
  Calories from Fat 5
Total Fat 1 g
  Saturated Fat 0 g
Cholesterol 0 mg
Sodium 314 mg
Total Carbohydrate 27 g
  Dietary Fiber 2 g
  Sugars 5 g
Protein 4 g

Grated Carrot-Raisin Salad

2 servings
Serving size: ½ recipe
Exchanges
1 Vegetable
1 Fruit
Calories 82
  Calories from Fat 3

Total Fat 0 g
  Saturated Fat 0 g
Cholesterol 0 mg
Sodium 174 mg
Total Carbohydrate 20 g
  Dietary Fiber 3 g
  Sugars 16 g
Protein 1 g

Chicken Cacciatore
4 servings
Serving size: ¼th recipe
Exchanges
3 Very Lean Meat
4 Vegetable
½ Fat
Calories 232
  Calories from Fat 55
Total Fat 6 g
  Saturated Fat 2 g
Cholesterol 72 mg
Sodium 581 mg
Total Carbohydrate 20 g
  Dietary Fiber 3 g
  Sugars 8 g
Protein 26 g

Shrimp Skewers
1 serving
Serving size: 3 skewers
Exchanges
4 Very Lean Meat
2 Vegetable
1 Fruit
Calories 243
  Calories from Fat 22
Total Fat 2 g
  Saturated Fat 0 g
Cholesterol 247 mg
Sodium 449 mg

Total Carbohydrate 27 g
  Dietary Fiber 4 g
  Sugars 20 g
Protein 30 g

Chicken Taco
12 servings
Serving size: 1 taco
Exchanges
1 Starch
3 Lean Meat
1 Vegetable
Calories 257
  Calories from Fat 66
Total Fat 7 g
  Saturated Fat 3 g
Cholesterol 56 mg
Sodium 481 mg
Total Carbohydrate 22 g
  Dietary Fiber 2 g
  Sugars 3 g
Protein 25 g

Pears Filled with Strawberry Cream Cheese
2 servings
Serving size: ½ recipe
Exchanges
1½ Fruit
2½ Fat
Calories 211
  Calories from Fat 112
Total Fat 12 g
  Saturated Fat 8 g
Cholesterol 40 mg
Sodium 239 mg
Total Carbohydrate 20 g
  Dietary Fiber 3 g
  Sugars 16 g
Protein 7 g

Kung Pao Chicken
4 servings
Serving size: $\frac{1}{4}$th recipe
Exchanges
$\frac{1}{2}$ Carbohydrate
3 Lean Meat
Calories 203
 Calories from Fat 104
Total Fat 12 g
 Saturated Fat 1 g
Cholesterol 53 mg
Sodium 358 mg
Total Carbohydrate 5 g
Dietary Fiber 0 g
Sugars 2 g
Protein 19 g

Nutty Rice Loaf
6 servings
Serving size: 1 slice
Exchanges
1 Starch
2 Medium-Fat Meat
Calories 217
 Calories from Fat 92
Total Fat 10 g
 Saturated Fat 3 g
Cholesterol 84 mg
Sodium 198 mg
Total Carbohydrate 19 g
 Dietary Fiber 3 g
 Sugars 3 g
Protein 14 g

Crab Cakes
4 servings
Serving size: 1 crab cake
Exchanges
2 Lean Meat
Calories 101
 Calories from Fat 36
Total Fat 4 g
 Saturated Fat 1 g

Cholesterol 101 mg
Sodium 305 mg
Total Carbohydrate 4 g
 Dietary Fiber 0 g
 Sugars 1 g
Protein 12 g

Greek Florentine Pizza
2 servings
Serving size: $\frac{1}{2}$ recipe
Exchanges
2 Starch
1 Medium-Fat Meat
2 Vegetable
1 Fat
Calories 332
 Calories from Fat 132
Total Fat 15 g
 Saturated Fat 6 g
Cholesterol 25 mg
Sodium 872 mg
Total Carbohydrate 38 g
 Dietary Fiber 5 g
 Sugars 7 g
Protein 14 g

Oven-Fried Fish
4 servings
Serving size: $\frac{1}{4}$th recipe
Exchanges
1 Starch
3 Very Lean Meat
$\frac{1}{2}$ Fat
Calories 212
 Calories from Fat 56
Total Fat 6 g
 Saturated Fat 0 g
Cholesterol 60 mg
Sodium 273 mg
Total Carbohydrate 14 g
 Dietary Fiber 0 g
 Sugars 2 g
Protein 24 g

Stuffed Zucchini

4 servings
Serving size: 2 halves
Exchanges
1 Starch
2 Medium-Fat Meat
4 Vegetable
1½ Fat
Calories 378
 Calories from Fat 168
Total Fat 19 g
 Saturated Fat 9 g
Cholesterol 145 mg
Sodium 869 mg
Total Carbohydrate 34 g
 Dietary Fiber 7 g
 Sugars 9 g
Protein 23 g

Chicken-Fried Steak with Pan Gravy

4 servings
Serving size: 1 serving
Exchanges
½ Starch
4 Lean Meat
Calories 265
 Calories from Fat 111
Total Fat 12 g
 Saturated Fat 2 g
Cholesterol 120 mg
Sodium 66 mg
Total Carbohydrate 11 g
 Dietary Fiber 0 g
 Sugars 2 g
Protein 26 g

Gelatin Fruit Parfait

1 serving
Serving size: 1 parfait
Exchanges
½ Fruit
½ Fat

Calories 61
 Calories from Fat 14
Total Fat 2 g
 Saturated Fat 1 g
Cholesterol 0 mg
Sodium 58 mg
Total Carbohydrate 10 g
 Dietary Fiber 1 g
 Sugars 7 g
Protein 2 g

Crustless Spinach Quiche

6 servings
Serving size: 1/6th recipe
Exchanges
1 Medium-Fat Meat
1 Vegetable
½ Fat
Calories 115
 Calories from Fat 58
Total Fat 6 g
 Saturated Fat 3 g
Cholesterol 153 mg
Sodium 180 mg
Total Carbohydrate 3 g
 Dietary Fiber 1 g
 Sugars 1 g
Protein 11 g

Crisp Red Cabbage

6 servings
Serving size: ½ cup
Exchanges
1 Carbohydrate
Calories 60
 Calories from Fat 3
Total Fat 0 g
 Saturated Fat 0 g
Cholesterol 0 mg
Sodium 109 mg

Total Carbohydrate 15 g
  Dietary Fiber 3 g
  Sugars 12 g
Protein 1 g

Sally's Hawaiian Chicken
8 servings
Serving size: ⅛th recipe
Exchanges
4 Very Lean Meat
1 Vegetable
½ Fruit
Calories 193
  Calories from Fat 27
Total Fat 3 g
  Saturated Fat 1 g
Cholesterol 68 mg
Sodium 468 mg
Total Carbohydrate 14 g
  Dietary Fiber 1 g
  Sugars 12 g
Protein 26 g

Vegetarian Lasagna
6 servings
Serving size: ⅙th recipe
Exchanges
3 Carbohydrate
2 Lean Meat
1½ Fat
Calories 406
  Calories from Fat 147
Total Fat 16 g
  Saturated Fat 4 g
Cholesterol 90 mg
Sodium 946 mg
Total Carbohydrate 44 g
  Dietary Fiber 7 g
  Sugars 11 g
Protein 25 g

Oven-Fried Chicken
2 servings
Serving size: ½ recipe
Exchanges
½ Starch
4 Very Lean Meat
1 Fat
Calories 225
  Calories from Fat 48
Total Fat 5 g
  Saturated Fat 2 g
Cholesterol 88 mg
Sodium 248 mg
Total Carbohydrate 8 g
  Dietary Fiber 0 g
  Sugars 1 g
Protein 34 g

Baked Apple I
2 servings
Serving size: 1/2 recipe
Exchanges
1 Fruit
Calories 66
  Calories from Fat 3
Total Fat 0 g
  Saturated Fat 0 g
Cholesterol 0 mg
Sodium 6 mg
Total Carbohydrate 17 g
  Dietary Fiber 3 g
  Sugars 14 g
Protein 0 g

Meat Loaf
6 servings
Serving size: ⅙th recipe
Exchanges
1 Starch
3 Medium-Fat Meat
½ Fat
Calories 333
  Calories from Fat 167

Total Fat 19 g
  Saturated Fat 7 g
Cholesterol 138 mg
Sodium 1045 mg
Total Carbohydrate 17 g
  Dietary Fiber 1 g
  Sugars 4 g
Protein 23 g

Grilled Pork Loin

4 servings
Serving size: ¼th recipe
Exchanges
3 Lean Meat
1 Vegetable
Calories 205
  Calories from Fat 73
Total Fat 8 g
  Saturated Fat 3 g
Cholesterol 78 mg
Sodium 66 mg
Total Carbohydrate 4 g
  Dietary Fiber 1 g
  Sugars 3 g
Protein 28 g

Orange Roughy Picante

4 servings
Serving size: ¼th recipe
Exchanges
3 Very Lean Meat
1 Vegetable
Calories 135
  Calories from Fat 31
Total Fat 3 g
  Saturated Fat 1 g
Cholesterol 32 mg
Sodium 589 mg
Total Carbohydrate 6 g
  Dietary Fiber 0 g
  Sugars 3 g
Protein 20 g

Sausage and Corn Bread Pie

4 servings
Serving size: ¼th recipe
Exchanges
2 Starch
2 Medium-Fat Meat
3 Vegetable
Calories 382
  Calories from Fat 96
Total Fat 11 g
  Saturated Fat 3 g
Cholesterol 113 mg
Sodium 1190 mg
Total Carbohydrate 44 g
  Dietary Fiber 7 g
  Sugars 10 g
Protein 29 g

Spinach Manicotti

5 servings
Serving size: ⅕th recipe
Exchanges
3 Carbohydrate
2 Very Lean Meat
Calories 305
  Calories from Fat 43
Total Fat 5 g
  Saturated Fat 2 g
Cholesterol 12 mg
Sodium 610 mg
Total Carbohydrate 48 g
  Dietary Fiber 7 g
  Sugars 8 g
Protein 24 g

Chicken Fajita

4 servings
Serving size: ½ cup
Exchanges
3 Lean Meat
1 Vegetable
Calories 205

Calories from Fat 74
Total Fat 8 g
  Saturated Fat 1 g
Cholesterol 68 mg
Sodium 289 mg
Total Carbohydrate 6 g
  Dietary Fiber 1 g
  Sugars 3 g
Protein 26 g

Grilled Tuna Steak
6 servings
Serving size: ⅙th recipe
Exchanges
4 Lean Meat
2 Fat
Calories 322
  Calories from Fat 178
Total Fat 20 g
  Saturated Fat 0 g
Cholesterol 56 mg
Sodium 450 mg
Total Carbohydrate 1 g
  Dietary Fiber 0 g
  Sugars 0 g
Protein 34 g

Turkey Polynesian
4 servings
Serving size: ¼th recipe
Exchanges
3 Very Lean Meat
2 Vegetable
1 Fruit
½ Fat
Calories 227
  Calories from Fat 38
Total Fat 4 g
  Saturated Fat 0 g
Cholesterol 53 mg
Sodium 116 mg

Total Carbohydrate 25 g
  Dietary Fiber 2 g
  Sugars 18 g
Protein 22 g

Noodle Pudding
4 servings
Serving size: ½ cup
Exchanges
1½ Carbohydrate
1 Fat
Calories 146
  Calories from Fat 42
Total Fat 5 g
  Saturated Fat 1 g
Cholesterol 67 mg
Sodium 21 mg
Total Carbohydrate 23 g
  Dietary Fiber 1 g
  Sugars 11 g
Protein 4 g

Grilled Lobster Tails
4 servings
Serving size: ¼th recipe
Exchanges
3 Very Lean Meat
1 Fat
Calories 138
  Calories from Fat 57
Total Fat 6 g
  Saturated Fat 4 g
Cholesterol 75 mg
Sodium 405 mg
Total Carbohydrate 1 g
  Dietary Fiber 0 g
  Sugars 1 g
Protein 17 g

Chicken with Sun-Dried Tomatoes
4 servings
Serving size: ¼th recipe

Exchanges
4 Very Lean Meat
½ Fat
Calories 177
  Calories from Fat 47
Total Fat 5 g
  Saturated Fat 0 g
Cholesterol 64 mg
Sodium 155 mg
Total Carbohydrate 3 g
  Dietary Fiber 1 g
  Sugars 2 g
Protein 27 g

Corn Soufflé
2 servings
Serving size: ½ recipe
Exchanges
2½ Starch
1 Medium-Fat Meat
½ Fat-Free Milk
1 Fat
Calories 348
  Calories from Fat 112
Total Fat 12 g
  Saturated Fat 4 g
Cholesterol 322 mg
Sodium 547 mg
Total Carbohydrate 45 g
  Dietary Fiber 4 g
  Sugars 12 g
Protein 19 g

Herbed Pork Kabobs
4 servings
Serving size: ¼th recipe
Exchanges
3 Lean Meat
1 Fat
Calories 216
  Calories from Fat 114
Total Fat 13 g
  Saturated Fat 3 g

Cholesterol 65 mg
Sodium 147 mg
Total Carbohydrate 0 g
  Dietary Fiber 0 g
  Sugars 0 g
Protein 24 g

Hearty Bean Stew
4 servings
Serving size: 1 cup
Exchanges
3 Starch
2 Vegetable
Calories 293
  Calories from Fat 19
Total Fat 2 g
  Saturated Fat 0 g
Cholesterol 0 mg
Sodium 743 mg
Total Carbohydrate 58 g
  Dietary Fiber 12 g
  Sugars 10 g
Protein 14 g

Pork Dijon
4 servings
Serving size: ¼th recipe
Exchanges
3 Lean Meat
Calories 173
  Calories from Fat 59
Total Fat 7 g
  Saturated Fat 2 g
Cholesterol 65 mg
Sodium 473 mg
Total Carbohydrate 3 g
  Dietary Fiber 0 g
  Sugars 1 g
Protein 25 g

Chicken Okra Gumbo
4 servings
Serving size: ¼th recipe

Exchanges
½ Starch
3 Very Lean Meat
2 Vegetable
1 Fat
Calories 259
  Calories from Fat 63
Total Fat 7 g
  Saturated Fat 1 g
Cholesterol 68 mg
Sodium 378 mg
Total Carbohydrate 18 g
  Dietary Fiber 4 g
  Sugars 5 g
Protein 29 g

Tamale Pie
4 servings
Serving size: ¼th recipe
Exchanges
3 Starch
1 Lean Meat
1 Vegetable
2 Fat
Calories 402
  Calories from Fat 150
Total Fat 17 g
  Saturated Fat 7 g
Cholesterol 107 mg
Sodium 762 mg
Total Carbohydrate 54 g
  Dietary Fiber 4 g
  Sugars 17 g
Protein 22 g

Bay Scallops Parmesan
4 servings
Serving size: ¼th recipe
Exchanges
3 Lean Meat
½ Fat
Calories 189
  Calories from Fat 89

Total Fat 10 g
  Saturated Fat 3 g
Cholesterol 55 mg
Sodium 465 mg
Total Carbohydrate 1 g
  Dietary Fiber 0 g
  Sugars 1 g
Protein 24 g

Chocolate Angel Food Cake
32 servings
Serving size: ½-inch serving
Exchanges
1 Carbohydrate
Calories 55
  Calories from Fat 2
Total Fat 0 g
  Saturated Fat 0 g
Cholesterol 0 mg
Sodium 119 mg
Total Carbohydrate 13 g
  Dietary Fiber 0 g
  Sugars 9 g
Protein 1 g

Seafood Boil
8 servings
Serving size: ⅛th recipe
Exchanges
1 Starch
2 Lean Meat
Calories 202
  Calories from Fat 50
Total Fat 6 g
  Saturated Fat 2 g
Cholesterol 119 mg
Sodium 953 mg
Total Carbohydrate 18 g
  Dietary Fiber 2 g
  Sugars 4 g
Protein 19 g

Mike's Veal

4 servings
Serving size: ¼th recipe
Exchanges
½ Starch
3 Lean Meat
1 Vegetable
Calories 228
   Calories from Fat 63
Total Fat 7 g
   Saturated Fat 2 g
Cholesterol 77 mg
Sodium 68 mg
Total Carbohydrate 13 g
   Dietary Fiber 3 g
   Sugars 4 g
Protein 27 g

Vegetable Stir-Fry

4 servings
Serving size: ¼th recipe
Exchanges
1 Starch
2 Lean Meat
1 Vegetable
2 Fat
Calories 305
   Calories from Fat 165
Total Fat 18 g
   Saturated Fat 7 g
Cholesterol 28 mg
Sodium 530 mg
Total Carbohydrate 19 g
   Dietary Fiber 2 g
   Sugars 7 g
Protein 23 g

Light and Creamy Yogurt Pie

8 servings
Serving size: ⅛th recipe
Exchanges
1½ Carbohydrate

1 Fat
Calories 156
   Calories from Fat 55
Total Fat 6 g
   Saturated Fat 2 g
Cholesterol 1 mg
Sodium 154 mg
Total Carbohydrate 21 g
   Dietary Fiber 1 g
   Sugars 11 g
Protein 2 g

New England Chicken Croquettes

4 servings
Serving size: 2 croquettes
Exchanges
1 Starch
4 Lean Meat
½ Fat
Calories 330
   Calories from Fat 131
Total Fat 15 g
   Saturated Fat 4 g
Cholesterol 169 mg
Sodium 648 mg
Total Carbohydrate 19 g
   Dietary Fiber 1 g
   Sugars 4 g
Protein 28 g

French Onion Soup

6 servings
Serving size: 1 cup
Exchanges
1 Starch
1 Vegetable
2 Fat
Calories 207
   Calories from Fat 82
Total Fat 9 g
   Saturated Fat 5 g
Cholesterol 23 mg

Sodium 863 mg
Total Carbohydrate 23 g
  Dietary Fiber 2 g
  Sugars 8 g
Protein 9 g

Hoppin' John
8 servings
Serving size: 1 cup
Exchanges
2 Starch
½ Fat
Calories 174
  Calories from Fat 23
Total Fat 3 g
  Saturated Fat 1 g
Cholesterol 3 mg
Sodium 52 mg
Total Carbohydrate 31 g
  Dietary Fiber 5 g
  Sugars 3 g
Protein 7 g

Seasoned Greens
8 servings
Serving size: ½ cup
Exchanges
1 Very Lean Meat
1 Vegetable
Calories 59
  Calories from Fat 17
Total Fat 2 g
  Saturated Fat 1 g
Cholesterol 18 mg
Sodium 23 mg
Total Carbohydrate 4 g
  Dietary Fiber 2 g
  Sugars 0 g
Protein 7 g

Salmon Loaf
4 servings
Serving size: 1 slice
Exchanges
1 Starch
3 Lean Meat
Calories 261
  Calories from Fat 90
Total Fat 10 g
  Saturated Fat 1 g
Cholesterol 169 mg
Sodium 765 mg
Total Carbohydrate 14 g
  Dietary Fiber 1 g
  Sugars 3 g
Protein 27 g

Picante Tofu and Rice
2 servings
Serving size: 1 recipe
Exchanges
3 Starch
1 Lean Meat
3 Vegetable
1 Fat
Calories 401
  Calories from Fat 93
Total Fat 10 g
  Saturated Fat 3 g
Cholesterol 10 mg
Sodium 971 mg
Total Carbohydrate 59 g
  Dietary Fiber 10 g
  Sugars 12 g
Protein 21 g

Broccoli Corn Chowder
16 servings
Serving size: 1 cup
Exchanges
1 Carbohydrate
½ Fat

Calories 101
   Calories from Fat 29
Total Fat 3 g
   Saturated Fat 1 g
Cholesterol 1 mg
Sodium 179 mg
Total Carbohydrate 15 g
   Dietary Fiber 2 g
   Sugars 4 g
Protein 4 g

Saucy Seafood Stir-Fry
4 servings
Serving size: ½th recipe
Exchanges
2 Lean Meat
1 Vegetable
Calories 133
   Calories from Fat 40
Total Fat 4 g
   Saturated Fat 0 g
Cholesterol 103 mg
Sodium 239 mg
Total Carbohydrate 6 g
   Dietary Fiber 2 g
   Sugars 3 g
Protein 17 g

Clam Sauce
5 servings
Serving size: 1 cup
Exchanges
1 Carbohydrate
3 Lean Meat
½ Fat
Calories 271
   Calories from Fat 114
Total Fat 13 g
   Saturated Fat 7 g
Cholesterol 85 mg
Sodium 605 mg
Total Carbohydrate 13 g
   Dietary Fiber 2 g

   Sugars 10 g
Protein 29 g

Chicken Curry
6 servings
Serving size: ⅙th recipe
Exchanges
½ Carbohydrate
3 Lean Meat
Calories 209
   Calories from Fat 73
Total Fat 8 g
   Saturated Fat 2 g
Cholesterol 65 mg
Sodium 94 mg
Total Carbohydrate 10 g
   Dietary Fiber 2 g
   Sugars 7 g
Protein 24 g

Prune-Stuffed Tenderloin
4 servings
Serving size: 1/4th recipe
Exchanges
1 Starch
3 Lean Meat
1 Fruit
Calories 306
   Calories from Fat 83
Total Fat 9 g
   Saturated Fat 2 g
Cholesterol 65 mg
Sodium 239 mg
Total Carbohydrate 31 g
   Dietary Fiber 4 g
   Sugars 16 g
Protein 27 g

Zucchini Lasagna
9 servings
Serving size: 1 piece
Exchanges

1½ Starch
2 Medium-Fat Meat
1 Vegetable
½ Fat
Calories 306
  Calories from Fat 111
Total Fat 12 g
  Saturated Fat 7 g
Cholesterol 81 mg
Sodium 506 mg
Total Carbohydrate 30 g
  Dietary Fiber 3 g
  Sugars 6 g
Protein 19 g

Brunswick Stew
4 servings
Serving size: 1½ cups
Exchanges
1½ Starch
2 Lean Meat
1 Vegetable
Calories 246
  Calories from Fat 50
Total Fat 6 g
  Saturated Fat 1 g
Cholesterol 45 mg
Sodium 842 mg
Total Carbohydrate 33 g
  Dietary Fiber 5 g
  Sugars 11 g
Protein 19 g

Chicken Ratatouille
4 servings
Serving size: ¼th recipe
Exchanges
4 Lean Meat
3 Vegetable
Calories 307
  Calories from Fat 87
Total Fat 10 g
  Saturated Fat 3 g

Cholesterol 93 mg
Sodium 152 mg
Total Carbohydrate 17 g
  Dietary Fiber 5 g
  Sugars 9 g
Protein 38 g

Yogurt Chicken Paprika
4 servings
Serving size: ¼th recipe
Exchanges
1 Carbohydrate
4 Very Lean Meat
1 Fat
Calories 257
  Calories from Fat 61
Total Fat 7 g
  Saturated Fat 3 g
Cholesterol 94 mg
Sodium 375 mg
Total Carbohydrate 12 g
  Dietary Fiber 1 g
  Sugars 8 g
Protein 35 g

Old-Fashioned Banana Pudding
6 servings
Serving size: ⅓ cup
Exchanges
1½ Carbohydrate
Calories 122
  Calories from Fat 14
Total Fat 2 g
  Saturated Fat 0 g
Cholesterol 6 mg
Sodium 287 mg
Total Carbohydrate 24 g
  Dietary Fiber 1 g
  Sugars 12 g
Protein 4 g

Stuffed Vegetarian Peppers

12 servings
Serving size: 1 pepper
Exchanges
1½ Starch
1 Vegetable
1 Fat
Calories 185
Calories from Fat 50
Total Fat 6 g
Saturated Fat 1 g
Cholesterol 0 mg
Sodium 9 mg
Total Carbohydrate 30 g
Dietary Fiber 6 g
Sugars 6 g
Protein 6 g

Italian Fruit Salad

6 servings
Serving size: ½ cup
Exchanges
1½ Fruit
Calories 77
Calories from Fat 4
Total Fat 0 g
Saturated Fat 0 g
Cholesterol 0 mg
Sodium 1 mg
Total Carbohydrate 20 g
Dietary Fiber 2 g
Sugars 15 g
Protein 1 g

Asian Chicken

4 servings
Serving size: ¼ cup
Exchanges
2 Lean Meat
3 Vegetable
1 Fat
Calories 226

Calories from Fat 84
Total Fat 9 g
Saturated Fat 2 g
Cholesterol 49 mg
Sodium 368 mg
Total Carbohydrate 13 g
Dietary Fiber 3 g
Sugars 7 g
Protein 17 g

Fruit Crisp

6 servings
Serving size: ¾ cup
Exchanges
1 Starch
1 Fruit
Calories 142
Calories from Fat 23
Total Fat 3 g
Saturated Fat 0 g
Cholesterol 0 mg
Sodium 33 mg
Total Carbohydrate 29 g
Dietary Fiber 4 g
Sugars 15 g
Protein 3 g

Porcupine Meatballs

2 servings
Serving size: 3 meatballs
Exchanges
1 Starch
2 Medium-Fat Meat
2 Vegetable
1 Fat
Calories 332
Calories from Fat 136
Total Fat 15 g
Saturated Fat 6 g
Cholesterol 71 mg
Sodium 802 mg
Total Carbohydrate 25 g
Dietary Fiber 2 g

Sugars 7 g
Protein 23 g

Baked Apple II
2 servings
Serving size: 1 apple
Exchanges
1 Fruit
1 Fat
Calories 105
Calories from Fat 38
Total Fat 4 g
Saturated Fat 1 g
Cholesterol 0 mg
Sodium 46 mg
Total Carbohydrate 18 g
Dietary Fiber 3 g
Sugars 15 g
Protein 0 g

Barbecued Chicken
2 servings
Serving size: ½ recipe
Exchanges
4 Lean Meat
Calories 199
Calories from Fat 75
Total Fat 8 g
Saturated Fat 2 g
Cholesterol 89 mg
Sodium 277 mg
Total Carbohydrate 3 g
Dietary Fiber 1 g
Sugars 2 g
Protein 27 g

Barbecue Sauce
18 servings
Serving size: ¼th cup
Exchanges
Free Food
Calories 14
Calories from Fat 1

Total Fat 0 g
Saturated Fat 0 g
Cholesterol 0 mg
Sodium 198 mg
Total Carbohydrate 3 g
Dietary Fiber 1 g
Sugars 2 g
Protein 0 g

Sally Lunn Peach Cake
12 servings
Serving size: 1 slice
Exchanges
2 Carbohydrate
2 Fat
Calories 212
Calories from Fat 91
Total Fat 10 g
Saturated Fat 0 g
Cholesterol 18 mg
Sodium 201 mg
Total Carbohydrate 27 g
Dietary Fiber 2 g
Sugars 10 g
Protein 4 g

Fish Creole
4 servings
Serving size: ¼th recipe
Exchanges
3 Lean Meat
1 Vegetable
Calories 205
Calories from Fat 78
Total Fat 9 g
Saturated Fat 1 g
Cholesterol 37 mg
Sodium 338 mg
Total Carbohydrate 7 g
Dietary Fiber 1 g
Sugars 4 g
Protein 25 g

Bok Choy Sauté

2 servings
Serving size: ½ recipe
Exchanges
3 Lean Meat
2 Vegetable
½ Fat
Calories 231
   Calories from Fat 101
Total Fat 11 g
   Saturated Fat 3 g
Cholesterol 65 mg
Sodium 359 mg
Total Carbohydrate 8 g
   Dietary Fiber 2 g
   Sugars 3 g
Protein 25 g

Black Bean Cakes

2 servings
Serving size: 2 cakes
Exchanges
2½ Starch
1 Very Lean Meat
1 Vegetable
2½ Fat
Calories 375
   Calories from Fat 146
Total Fat 16 g
   Saturated Fat 4 g
Cholesterol 107 mg
Sodium 168 mg
Total Carbohydrate 43 g
   Dietary Fiber 11 g
   Sugars 7 g
Protein 16 g

Cilantro Salsa

4 servings
Serving size: ½ cup
Exchanges
1 Vegetable
Calories 36

   Calories from Fat 3
Total Fat 0 g
   Saturated Fat 0 g
Cholesterol 0 mg
Sodium 9 mg
Total Carbohydrate 8 g
   Dietary Fiber 2 g
   Sugars 5 g
Protein 1 g

Jambalaya

4 servings
Serving size: 1½ cups
Exchanges
2 Starch
2 Lean Meat
3 Vegetable
Calories 338
   Calories from Fat 61
Total Fat 7 g
   Saturated Fat 0 g
Cholesterol 152 mg
Sodium 851 mg
Total Carbohydrate 43 g
   Dietary Fiber 5 g
   Sugars 9 g
Protein 27 g

Hawaiian Kabobs

4 servings
Serving size: 2 skewers
Exchanges
3 Lean Meat
2 Vegetable
1 Fruit
Calories 277
   Calories from Fat 94
Total Fat 10 g
   Saturated Fat 1 g
Cholesterol 60 mg
Sodium 213 mg
Total Carbohydrate 22 g
   Dietary Fiber 4 g

Sugars 15 g
Protein 25 g

Apricot-Glazed Ham
4 servings
Serving size: ½ recipe
Exchanges
3 Very Lean Meat
1 Fruit
Calories 161
Calories from Fat 33
Total Fat 4 g
Saturated Fat 1 g
Cholesterol 38 mg
Sodium 1082 mg
Total Carbohydrate 14 g
Dietary Fiber 1 g
Sugars 12 g
Protein 17 g

Lightly Scalloped Potatoes
8 servings
Serving size: ½ cup
Exchanges
1½ Starch
½ Fat
Calories 140
Calories from Fat 28
Total Fat 3 g
Saturated Fat 2 g
Cholesterol 10 mg
Sodium 339 mg
Total Carbohydrate 21 g
Dietary Fiber 2 g
Sugars 5 g
Protein 9 g

Raspberry-Orange Gelatin Supreme
6 servings
Serving size: ¾ cup
Exchanges

1 Fruit
Calories 66
Calories from Fat 2
Total Fat 0 g
Saturated Fat 0 g
Cholesterol 0 mg
Sodium 79 mg
Total Carbohydrate 15 g
Dietary Fiber 0 g
Sugars 4 g
Protein 2 g

Seafood Casserole
6 servings
Serving size: 1 cup
Exchanges
1½ Starch
3 Very Lean Meat
½ Fat
Calories 247
Calories from Fat 48
Total Fat 5 g
Saturated Fat 2 g
Cholesterol 161 mg
Sodium 360 mg
Total Carbohydrate 20 g
Dietary Fiber 3 g
Sugars 4 g
Protein 29 g

Tofu-Vegetable Stir-Fry
4 servings
Serving size: 2 cups
Exchanges
1 Medium-Fat Meat
2 Vegetable
1½ Fat
Calories 189
Calories from Fat 114
Total Fat 13 g
Saturated Fat 3 g
Cholesterol 0 mg
Sodium 347 mg

Total Carbohydrate 14 g
  Dietary Fiber 4 g
  Sugars 8 g
Protein 8 g

Pineapple-Oatmeal Cake
9 servings
Serving size: 1/9 recipe
Exchanges
1 Starch
1/2 Fruit
1 Fat
Calories 143
  Calories from Fat 46
Total Fat 5 g
  Saturated Fat 1 g
Cholesterol 48 mg
Sodium 138 mg
Total Carbohydrate 20 g
  Dietary Fiber 3 g
  Sugars 8 g
Protein 5 g

Polenta
4 servings
Serving size: 2 wedges
Exchanges
2 1/2 Starch
Calories 189
  Calories from Fat 6
Total Fat 1 g
  Saturated Fat 0 g
Cholesterol 0 mg
Sodium 481 mg
Total Carbohydrate 37 g
  Dietary Fiber 3 g
  Sugars 1 g
Protein 7 g

Marinara Sauce
4 servings
Serving size: 1/4 cup
Exchanges

1 Vegetable
Calories 29
  Calories from Fat 1
Total Fat 0 g
  Saturated Fat 0 g
Cholesterol 0 mg
Sodium 311 mg
Total Carbohydrate 7 g
  Dietary Fiber 1 g
  Sugars 5 g
Protein 1 g

Bean Burger
8 servings
Serving size: 1 burger
Exchanges
1 1/2 Starch
Calories 122
  Calories from Fat 16
Total Fat 2 g
  Saturated Fat 1 g
Cholesterol 4 mg
Sodium 308 mg
Total Carbohydrate 22 g
  Dietary Fiber 3 g
  Sugars 3 g
Protein 6 g

Breakfast in a Cookie
21 servings
Serving size: 2 cookies
Exchanges
1/2 Starch
1/2 Fruit
1/2 Fat
Calories 103
  Calories from Fat 25
Total Fat 3 g
  Saturated Fat 1 g
Cholesterol 10 mg
Sodium 108 mg
Total Carbohydrate 18 g
  Dietary Fiber 2 g

Sugars 9 g
Protein 3 g

Chicken Casserole
4 servings
Serving size: 1 cup
Exchanges
½ Carbohydrate
1 Lean Meat
Calories 103
Calories from Fat 36
Total Fat 4 g
Saturated Fat 1 g
Cholesterol 23 mg
Sodium 88 mg
Total Carbohydrate 7 g
Dietary Fiber 1 g
Sugars 3 g
Protein 10 g

Hearty Onion-Garlic Soup
4 servings
Serving size: 1½ cups
Exchanges
1 Starch
3 Vegetable
1½ Fat
Calories 217
Calories from Fat 72
Total Fat 8 g
Saturated Fat 1 g
Cholesterol 0 mg
Sodium 1015 mg
Total Carbohydrate 34 g
Dietary Fiber 6 g
Sugars 17 g
Protein 6 g

Spinach-Stuffed Chicken Breasts
4 servings
Serving size: ¼th recipe

Exchanges
5 Very Lean Meat
½ Fat
Calories 211
Calories from Fat 50
Total Fat 6 g
Saturated Fat 2 g
Cholesterol 96 mg
Sodium 160 mg
Total Carbohydrate 2 g
Dietary Fiber 1 g
Sugars 1 g
Protein 36 g

Tortellini Primavera
1 serving
Serving size: 1 recipe
Exchanges
2½ Starch
1 Medium-Fat Meat
2 Vegetable
½ Fat-Free Milk
2 Fat
Calories 460
Calories from Fat 146
Total Fat 16 g
Saturated Fat 6 g
Cholesterol 52 mg
Sodium 678 mg
Total Carbohydrate 55 g
Dietary Fiber 4 g
Sugars 13 g
Protein 27 g

Dahl
2 servings
Serving size: ½ recipe
Exchanges
3 Starch
2 Very Lean Meat
1 Vegetable
½ Fat
Calories 349

240

Calories from Fat 54
Total Fat 6 g
  Saturated Fat 0 g
Cholesterol 0 mg
Sodium 11 mg
Total Carbohydrate 55 g
  Dietary Fiber 20 g
  Sugars 10 g
Protein 22 g

Macedonia Fruit Cup
10 servings
Serving size: ½ cup
Exchanges
1 Fruit
Calories 61
  Calories from Fat 3
Total Fat 0 g
  Saturated Fat 0 g
Cholesterol 0 mg
Sodium 1 mg
Total Carbohydrate 15 g
  Dietary Fiber 2 g
  Sugars 12 g
Protein 1 g

Fruit Punch
12 servings
Serving size: ½ cup
Exchanges
1 Fruit
Calories 54
  Calories from Fat 1
Total Fat 0 g
  Saturated Fat 0 g
Cholesterol 0 mg
Sodium 5 mg
Total Carbohydrate 13 g
  Dietary Fiber 0 g
  Sugars 12 g
Protein 0 g

Frosty Grapes
4 servings
Serving size: ¼th recipe
Exchanges
1 Fruit
Calories 68
  Calories from Fat 5
Total Fat 1 g
  Saturated Fat 0 g
Cholesterol 0 mg
Sodium 58 mg
Total Carbohydrate 16 g
  Dietary Fiber 1 g
  Sugars 12 g
Protein 2 g

Chocolate-Flavored Syrup
15 servings
Serving size: 2 Tbsp.
Exchanges
Free Food
Calories 10
  Calories from Fat 4
Total Fat 0 g
  Saturated Fat 0 g
Cholesterol 0 mg
Sodium 39 mg
Total Carbohydrate 2 g
  Dietary Fiber 1 g
  Sugars 1 g
Protein 1 g

Strawberry Whip
4 servings
Serving size: ¾ cup
Exchanges
½ Carbohydrate
Calories 47
  Calories from Fat 1
Total Fat 0 g
  Saturated Fat 0 g
Cholesterol 1 mg

Sodium 100 mg
Total Carbohydrate 7 g
  Dietary Fiber 1 g
  Sugars 6 g
Protein 5 g

Black Bean Dip
6 servings
Serving size: ⅓ cup
Exchanges
1 Starch
½ Fat
Calories 104
  Calories from Fat 30
Total Fat 3 g
  Saturated Fat 1 g
Cholesterol 0 mg
Sodium 64 mg
Total Carbohydrate 15 g
  Dietary Fiber 5 g
  Sugars 3 g
Protein 5 g

Vanilla Milkshake
1 serving
Serving size: 1½ cups
Exchanges
2 Carbohydrate
Calories 176
  Calories from Fat 4
Total Fat 0 g
  Saturated Fat 0 g
Cholesterol 4 mg
Sodium 191 mg
Total Carbohydrate 30 g
  Dietary Fiber 0 g
  Sugars 14 g
Protein 12 g

Peachy Whole-Grain Cookie
30 servings
Serving size: 1 cookie
Exchanges
1 Carbohydrate
Calories 68
  Calories from Fat 21
Total Fat 2 g
  Saturated Fat 0 g
Cholesterol 0 mg
Sodium 78 mg
Total Carbohydrate 11 g
  Dietary Fiber 1 g
  Sugars 7 g
Protein 1 g

Oklahoma Bean Salad
10 servings
Serving size: ½ cup
Exchanges
1½ Starch
Calories 107
  Calories from Fat 6
Total Fat 1 g
  Saturated Fat 0 g
Cholesterol 0 mg
Sodium 346 mg
Total Carbohydrate 20 g
  Dietary Fiber 5 g
  Sugars 5 g
Protein 6 g

Index

This index groups the recipes found in *Magic Menus* by main ingredient or type of food, for instance, chicken or dessert. There is also a heading called Potpourri, where you will find unique recipes, such as breakfast foods, dips, and sandwiches.

BEANS

Bean Burgers, 186
Black Bean Cakes, 174
Black Bean Dip, 204
Hoppin' John, 148
Hummus with Red Pepper, 92
Oklahoma Bean Salad, 209
Pintos and Potatoes, 86
Spanish Garbanzo Beans, 80
Spicy Black-Eyed Peas, 68

BEEF

Chicken-Fried Steak with Pan
   Gravy, 112
Creamed Chipped Beef over
   Toast, 34
Meat Loaf, 122
Mike's Veal, 143
Porcupine Meatballs, 168
Sloppy Joes, 63
Tamale Pie, 139

BREADS, MUFFINS, & PANCAKES

Angel Biscuits, 35
Apple-Raisin Muffins, 33
Atomic Muffin, 48
Breakfast in a Cookie, 187
Fluffy High-Fiber, Low-Fat
   Pancakes, 39
Granola Pancakes, 47
Iowa Corn Pancakes, 42
Johnnycake, 46
Peachy Whole-Grain Cookies,
   208
Peanut Butter and Jelly
   Muffins, 41
Pizza Muffins, 76
Scones, 28

Strawberry Shortcake, 21
Sugar-Free Blueberry Muffins, 25
Sweet Potato–Raisin Cookies, 43
Whole-Grain Muffins, 95
Whole-Wheat Currant Scones,
   50

CHICKEN & TURKEY

Asian Chicken, 166
Barbecued Chicken, 170
Brunswick Stew, 160
Chicken Cacciatore, 102
Chicken Casserole, 188
Chicken Curry, 155
Chicken Fajita, 127
Chicken Okra Gumbo, 138
Chicken Ratatouille, 161
Chicken Tacos, 104
Chicken with Sun-Dried
   Tomatoes, 132
Frogmore Stew, 142
Hawaiian Kabobs, 177
Kung Pao Chicken, 106
New England Chicken
   Croquettes, 146
Oven-Fried Chicken, 120
Sally's Hawaiian Chicken, 117
Spicy Turkey Loaf, 75
Spinach-Stuffed Chicken
   Breasts, 190
Turkey Polynesian, 129
Turkey-Squash Casserole, 78
Yogurt Chicken Paprika, 162

DESSERTS

Baked Apple I, 121
Baked Apple II, 169
Baked Rice Pudding, 44

Breakfast Parfait, 23
Chocolate Angel Food Cake, 141
Frosty Grapes, 198
Fruit Crisp, 167
Gelatin Fruit Parfait, 114
Graham Pudding Sandwiches, 29
Italian Fruit Salad, 165
Light and Creamy Yogurt Pie, 145
Low-Fat Lemon Cheesecake, 89
Old-Fashioned Banana Pudding, 163
Peachy Whole-Grain Cookie, 208
Pears Filled with Strawberry Cream Cheese, 105
Pineapple-Oatmeal Cake, 183
Raspberry-Orange Gelatin Supreme, 180
Sally Lunn Peach Cake, 171
Strawberry Shortcake, 21
Strawberry Whip, 200

DRINKS
Breakfast Blender Drink, 30
Café Mocha, 192
Commuter Breakfast, 23
Fruit Punch, 197
Strawberry Blender Drink, 18
Vanilla Milkshake, 207

FRUIT
Baked Apple I, 121
Baked Apple II, 169
Frosty Grapes, 198
Fruit Crisp, 167
Fruit Punch, 197
Gelatin Fruit Parfait, 114
Grapefruit Grand, 37
Italian Fruit Salad, 165
Macedonia Fruit Cup, 196
Old-Fashioned Banana Pudding, 163
Pears Filled with Strawberry Cream Cheese, 105

Strawberry Shortcake, 21
Strawberry Whip, 200

PORK
Apricot-Glazed Ham, 178
Bok Choy Sauté, 173
Grilled Pork Loin, 123
Herbed Pork Kabobs, 135
Hoppin' John, 148
Jambalaya, 176
Low Country Grits and Sausage, 45
Pork Dijon, 137
Prune-Stuffed Tenderloin, 156
Sausage and Corn Bread Pie, 125
Schinkennudelin, 81

POTPOURRI
Barbecue Sauce, 170
Black Bean Dip, 204
Chocolate-Flavored Syrup, 199
Cilantro Salsa, 175
Cinnamon Tortilla Pocket, 22
Crunchy Granola, 31
Easy Spud Breakfast, 27
English Muffin Pizza Melt, 64
French Dressing, 59
Graham Pudding Sandwiches, 29
Greek Florentine Pizza, 109
Oatmeal-Wheatena Porridge with Banana and Walnuts, 49
Ricotta Cheese Spread, 26
Schinkennudelin, 81
Spanish Omelette, 36
Submarine Sandwich, 66
Tortilla Ranch Style, 65
Veggie Pizza, 71
Whole-Wheat Pizza, 60

SALADS
Bean Salad, 94
Caesar Salad, 84
Grated Carrot-Raisin Salad, 97
Italian Fruit Salad, 165
Light Spinach Salad, 72
Noodle Supreme Salad, 61

244

Oklahoma Bean Salad, 209
Seven-Layer Salad, 83
Shrimp and Pea Salad, 88
Rigatoni Salad, 96

SEAFOOD
Bay Scallops Parmesan, 140
Clam Sauce, 154
Crab Cakes, 108
Crunchy Tuna Cheese Melt, 69
Fish Creole, 172
Grilled Lobster Tails, 131
Grilled Tuna Steak, 128
Jambalaya, 176
Orange Roughy Picante, 124
Oven-Fried Fish, 110
Pan-Broiled Shrimp, 79
Salmon Loaf, 150
Saucy Seafood Stir-Fry, 153
Seafood Boil, 142
Seafood Casserole, 181
Shrimp Skewers, 103

SIDE DISHES
Cheesy Grits, 32
Corn Soufflé, 134
Crisp Red Cabbage, 116
Cucumbers with Dill Dressing, 93
Fiesta Rice, 77
Lightly Scalloped Potatoes, 179
Mastokhiar, 87
Noodle Pudding, 130
Pintos and Potatoes, 86
Seasoned Greens, 149
Spanish Garbanzo Beans, 80
Spicy Black-Eyed Peas, 68

SOUPS
Black Bean Soup, 62
Broccoli-Corn Chowder, 152
Brunswick Stew, 160
Fast Corn Chowder, 70
French Onion Soup, 147
Gazpacho, 73
Hearty Bean Stew, 136
Hearty Onion-Garlic Soup, 189
Lentil-Veggie Soup, 82
Minestrone, 67
Southwestern Veggie Soup, 90

VEGGIE ENTREES
Bean Burgers, 186
Black Bean Cakes, 174
Broccoli Quiche, 38
Broiled Open-Faced Vegetarian Sandwich, 74
Crustless Spinach Quiche, 115
Dahl, 192
Hearty Bean Stew, 136
Nutty Rice Loaf, 107
Picante Tofu and Rice, 151
Spinach Manicotti, 126
Stuffed Vegetarian Peppers, 164
Stuffed Zucchini, 111
Tofu Garden Quiche, 40
Tofu-Vegetable Stir-Fry, 182
Tortellini Primavera, 191
Vegetable Stir-Fry, 144
Vegetarian Lasagna, 118
Zucchini Lasagna, 158

About the American Diabetes Association

The American Diabetes Association is the nation's leading voluntary health organization supporting diabetes research, information, and advocacy. Its mission is to prevent and cure diabetes and to improve the lives of all people affected by diabetes. The American Diabetes Association is the leading publisher of comprehensive diabetes information. Its huge library of practical and authoritative books for people with diabetes covers every aspect of self-care—cooking and nutrition, fitness, weight control, medications, complications, emotional issues, and general self-care.

To order American Diabetes Association books: Call 1-800-232-6733. http://store.diabetes.org [Note: there is no need to use www when typing this particular Web address]

To join the American Diabetes Association: Call 1-800-806-7801. www.diabetes.org/membership

For more information about diabetes or ADA programs and services: Call 1-800-342-2383. E-mail: Customerservice@diabetes.org

To locate an ADA/NCQA Recognized Provider of quality diabetes care in your area: www.ncqa.org/dprp/

To find an ADA Recognized Education Program in your area: Call 1-888-232-0822. www.diabetes.org/recognition/education.asp

To join the fight to increase funding for diabetes research, end discrimination, and improve insurance coverage: Call 1-800-342-2383. www.diabetes.org/advocacy

To find out how you can get involved with the programs in your community: Call 1-800-342-2383. See below for program Web addresses.

- *American Diabetes Month:* Educational activities aimed at those diagnosed with diabetes—month of November. www.diabetes.org/ADM
- *American Diabetes Alert:* Annual public awareness campaign to find the undiagnosed—held the fourth Tuesday in March. www.diabetes.org/alert
- *The Diabetes Assistance & Resources Program (DAR):* diabetes awareness program targeted to the Latino community. www.diabetes.org/DAR
- *African American Program:* diabetes awareness program targeted to the African American community. www.diabetes.org/africanamerican
- *Awakening the Spirit: Pathways to Diabetes Prevention & Control:* diabetes awareness program targeted to the Native American community. www.diabetes.org/awakening

To find out about an important research project regarding type 2 diabetes: www.diabetes.org/ada/research.asp

To obtain information on making a planned gift or charitable bequest: Call 1-888-700-7029. www.diabetes.org/ada/plan.asp

To make a donation or memorial contribution: Call 1-800-342-2383. www.diabetes.org/ada/cont.asp